Disability in Higher Education

Disability in Higher Education

Investigating identity, stigma, and disclosure amongst academics

Gayle Brewer

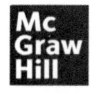

Mc Graw Hill

Open University Press

Open University Press
McGraw Hill
8th Floor, 338 Euston Road
London
England
NW1 3BH

email: enquiries@openup.co.uk
world wide web: www.openup.co.uk

First edition published 2022

Copyright © Open International Publishing Limited, 2022

All rights reserved. Except for the quotation of short passages for the purposes of criticism and review, no part of this publication may be reproduced, stored in a retrieval system, or transmitted, in any form or by any means, electronic, mechanical, photocopying, recording or otherwise, without the prior written permission of the publisher or a licence from the Copyright Licensing Agency Limited. Details of such licences (for reprographic reproduction) may be obtained from the Copyright Licensing Agency Ltd of Saffron House, 6–10 Kirby Street, London EC1N 8TS.

A catalogue record of this book is available from the British Library

ISBN-13: 9780335250318
ISBN-10: 0335250319
eISBN: 9780335250608

Library of Congress Cataloging-in-Publication Data
CIP data applied for

Typeset by Transforma Pvt. Ltd., Chennai, India

Fictitious names of companies, products, people, characters and/or data that may be used herein (in case studies or in examples) are not intended to represent any real individual, company, product or event.

Praise page

"*Gayle Brewer's Disability in Higher Education is a clear, concise, accessible yet detailed exploration of the realities of disability in the Academy. Gayle Brewer provides a carefully crafted, comprehensive and multifaceted examination of the various layers and textures of the lives of disabled academics. Far from the traditional, simplified, and tragic overcoming narrative, the author presents unflinching perspectives drawn from daily life as it is.*"

Nancy Hansen, Professor, Director Disability Studies,
University of Manitoba, Canada

"*I am proud to endorse Dr Brewer's much-anticipated work on Disability in Higher Education. As institutes of knowledge, discovery and innovation, universities should be inspiring the rest of society to create an environment where everyone can thrive, whether students or employees. However, this book exposes the barriers, stigma and discrimination that disabled academics face daily, overtly and covertly, in a profession we are passionate about. Dr Brewer demonstrates the pivotal concepts of Nothing About Us Without Us and real lived experience by including powerful quotes from disabled academics she interviewed. Recommendations are presented seeking to redress systemic ableism and promote equality, diversity, inclusion, and accessibility in Higher Education.*"

Dr Hamied Haroon, Chair, National Association of
Disabled Staff Networks (NADSN)

*For those who fight every day to be accepted, to be included, and to be valued.
We exist, we contribute, we matter.*

Contents

Preface xii
Acknowledgements xiii
Introduction xiv

1 REPRESENTING DISABILITY 1
    Media representations of disability 1
        Disability drag 2
        Advertising 3
        Mental health 4
    Disability-focused media and social media 5
    Language 7
    Models of disability 8
        The medical model 8
        The social model 9
        Alternative models 10
    Conducting research: nothing about us without us 11
    Summary 12
    Sport and the supercrip stereotype 13
    Teachers and academics in the media 14

2 STIGMA AND DISCRIMINATION 16
    Defining stigma 16
    Stigma and disability 18
    Conditions susceptible to stigma 19
        Schizophrenia 19
        HIV/AIDS 20
    Workplace discrimination 21
        Workplace accommodations 22
        Perceived competence 24
    Academia, stigma, and discrimination 24
    Summary 27
    Measuring attitudes towards disability 27
    Sexual orientation and stigma 28

3 ACADEMIC CULTURE AND CONTEXT 30
    Academic culture 30
        The emergence of Neoliberal ideology 31
        Performance metrics 32
        Giroux: Challenging the Neoliberal agenda 32
    The academic role 33

	Ableism and disability in academia	35
	Adjustments and accommodations	38
	Academia and the COVID-19 pandemic	40
	Summary	42
4	**INVISIBLE DISABILITIES AND THE DECISION TO DISCLOSE**	**43**
	Invisible disabilities and identity	43
	Self-disclosure	45
	Factors influencing the decision to disclose	46
	Types of disclosure	48
	Non-disclosure and passing	49
	Responses to disclosure	50
	Summary	52
	Status and reputation	53
5	**EXPERIENCES OF DISABLED ACADEMICS**	**54**
	Identity, stigma, and disclosure	54
	The academic environment	55
	Autism	56
	Strengths rather than deficits	57
	Dyslexia	58
	Dyslexic teachers and academics	59
	Mental health conditions	61
	Autoethnographic accounts	63
	Musculoskeletal disorders	63
	Energy-limiting conditions	65
	COVID-19	67
	Summary	68
6	**PERCEPTIONS OF DISABLED ACADEMICS AND DISABILITY**	**69**
	Student evaluations	69
	Academic role models	71
	Disabled identity and disability pride	73
	Non-disabled students	74
	Academic experiences and disclosure	75
	'Faking it' and perceived malingering	76
	Summary	80
	Challenging perceptions: Disability simulation	80
7	**ADVICE AND GUIDANCE**	**83**
	The academic role	83
	Promotion	84
	Part-time roles and precarious contracts	85
	Research publication, funding, and assessment	86
	Publication	86
	Funding	87
	Assessment and metrics	88
	Accommodation and inclusive design	89
	Securing accommodations, diagnosis, and disclosure	91
	Funding accommodations	92

Specific impairments and disciplines	93
Academic conferences and events	95
Conference accommodation and accessibility	96
Mentoring, support, and disabled staff networks	98
Education and training	99
COVID-19 and remote working	101
Summary	104
Additional sources of interest	104
Conclusion	105
References	106
Index	129

Preface

Higher education constitutes a challenging and competitive environment, with academia increasingly characterized by long working hours and the use of standardized metrics to monitor and evaluate performance. This environment is especially problematic for those with additional needs or responsibilities, such as carers and academics with disabilities. This book provides an insight into disability and ableism in higher education, placing particular emphasis on the experiences of academics who are themselves disabled. Indeed, it has been written in large part as a response to my own experience as a disabled academic and engagement with the disabled academic community.

The book covers a range of issues, including the stigma associated with disability, workplace discrimination, the decision to disclose a disability, and access to workplace accommodations. Recommendations to address the structural and operational issues that systematically disadvantage disabled academics are provided throughout the book, with one chapter dedicated to this issue. Overall, the book aims to inform and advise those interested in disability within higher education. It is of relevance not only to those who identify as disabled but also to senior management, policymakers and students of disability studies or education.

Acknowledgements

This book could not have been written without the support of the disabled academics interviewed. I will be forever grateful for their openness and generosity, providing their time to discuss their personal lived experience as disabled academics. I am also grateful for the support and guidance of people at the Open University Press, especially Zoë Osman, Eleanor Christie, and Laura Pacey. Finally, I would like to thank my family and friends for their support. I could not have completed this without them.

Introduction

Disabled people face a number of challenges, including stigma, accessibility, and workplace discrimination. Despite this, there is little recognition of the lived experience of disabled academics. It is important to acknowledge the presence and value of disabled academics and to address the systemic and structural issues that serve to disadvantage disabled faculty. This book contributes to an emerging literature that recognizes disability within higher education, with the intention to increase the accessibility and diversity of academia. Note that in this text, disability refers to a physical or mental impairment that has a substantial and long-term negative effect on a person's ability to complete routine activities and both identity-first (disabled academics) and person-first (academics with disabilities) language is adopted throughout.

Chapter 1, *Representing Disability*, considers the broader issues that impact on disabled people. In particular, the chapter outlines representations of disability, including stereotyped depictions of disabled people as a threat to society or a burden to others. The positive impact of specialist media created by people with disabilities and social media is also discussed. The chapter introduces models that frame our understanding of disability. Particular emphasis is placed on the medical and social models, although alternative models (e.g. the capability and affirmation models) are introduced. Finally, the chapter addresses the importance of conducting research *with* not *on* disabled people and recognizing the extent to which the voices of disabled people are often marginalized or dismissed.

Chapter 2, *Stigma and Discrimination*, focuses on the stigma, prejudice, and discrimination experienced by disabled people. A range of stigma types (e.g. self-stigma and label avoidance) are discussed. Some impairments are particularly susceptible to stigma and discrimination. The chapter addresses two especially stigmatized conditions (schizophrenia and HIV/AIDS) and factors impacting on the level of stigma experienced (e.g. concealability and disruptiveness). The chapter considers the experience and impact of workplace discrimination, with discrimination apparent at each stage of the employment process (e.g. recruitment, promotion, and retention). Particular emphasis is placed on prejudice in relation to perceived competence and access to the workplace accommodations that support disabled employees.

Chapter 3, *Academic Culture and Context*, focuses on the specific issues experienced by disabled people based within higher education. The most problematic aspects of the prevailing Neoliberal culture are highlighted. In particular, the chapter discusses the use of performance metrics, excessive workloads, long working hours, and precarious contracts. The impact of ableism in academia is discussed together with the experience of requesting workplace accommodations.

Chapter 4, *Invisible Disabilities and the Decision to Disclose*, focuses on impairments that may not be immediately apparent (e.g. arthritis, endometriosis, fibromyalgia). Those without visible signals of disability (such as mobility aids) are typically assumed to be non-disabled. As a consequence, people with invisible impairments must decide whether to self-disclose their condition (increasing the likelihood of stigma and discrimination) or "pass" as a person without disabilities (limiting access to support and workplace accommodations). The chapter considers the experience of invisible impairments and the development of a disabled identity. The decision to disclose a disability and factors that influence an individual's decision to self-disclose an invisible disability are also discussed.

Chapter 5, *Experiences of Disabled Academics*, focuses on personal experiences of disability within higher education. The chapter discusses shared personal experiences of stigma, disabled identity, and disclosure. The impact of the academic environment (e.g. excessive workloads) is also addressed. Recognizing the issues that may arise in response to specific conditions, the chapter looks at experiences of autism, dyslexia, mental health conditions, musculoskeletal disorders, and energy-limiting conditions in particular depth.

Chapter 6, *Perceptions of Disabled Academics and Disability*, considers disabled and non-disabled student perceptions of disability. These perceptions have important ramifications for the progression of disabled academics (e.g. student evaluations informing promotion criteria) and may, therefore, impact on the decision to disclose a disability. The presence of disabled academics may also impact on the student experience. For example, disabled faculty serve as role models, influencing student attitudes and behaviour. Their presence may be especially important for students with disabilities, supporting the development of a positive disabled identity.

Chapter 7, *Advice and Guidance*, provides recommendations to address the structural and operational issues that systematically disadvantage disabled academics. Recommendations are targeted at university management, recognizing the additional labour that is already undertaken by disabled faculty to obtain accommodations, etc. The advice and guidance provided in the chapter focuses on the academic role (e.g. excessive workloads and precarious contracts), accommodations (e.g. inclusive design and the process of disclosure), and support available (e.g. mentoring and disabled staff networks).

Throughout, I have tried to prioritize the lived experience of disabled academics and amplify the voices of those with disabilities. Therefore, the book is informed not only by existing research literature and my own experience as a disabled academic, but by a series of individual interviews conducted with disabled faculty in October and November 2020 and May 2021. I will be forever grateful for the openness and generosity of those interviewed, who gave their valuable time to discuss their personal experience as disabled academics. This book would not exist without their contribution. To clearly differentiate between quotations originating from existing research and quotations from interviews that I conducted directly with disabled faculty, quotations from interviews that I personally conducted have been italicized.

1 Representing disability

In order to understand the experience of disabled academics, it is important to consider broader issues that impact on those with disabilities. In particular, it is important to understand common conceptualizations of disability and the way in which people with disabilities are represented. For many people, the media is the primary, or indeed only, source of information about disability or specific impairments. Hence, the media has the potential to create a positive and respectful – or negative and hostile – environment for disabled people. Furthermore, a range of models have been developed with different approaches to disability and recommendations for measures that should be taken to support the disabled community. These models provide an important insight into the treatment of disabled people, disabled identity, and campaigns coordinated by disabled activists. Therefore, this chapter will provide an overview of media representations of disability and models of disability.

Media representations of disability

> I believe movies are the most powerful medium for change on earth. They are also a powerful medium for institutionalizing complacency, oppression, and reaction. (Walker, 1996, p. 282)

Many people have little direct interaction with disabled people or limited opportunities to learn about specific conditions. Indeed, for many people, the media is their primary source of information about such subjects. As a consequence, the media has a powerful impact on their understanding of disability. As summarized by Safran (2001), "While movies entertain, they simultaneously provide viewers with information about disabilities, and, through the filmmaker's lens, they project representations of how individuals fit into a nation's social and political landscape" (p. 223). Disability is, however, often portrayed by the media in a negative or stereotyped manner.

Nelson (2000) identifies six common disability-related stereotypes: the disabled person as (1) victim, (2) hero, (3) a threat, (4) unable to adjust, (5) a burden, and (6) better off dead. The victim stereotype views disability as a tragedy and those who are disabled in need of external support. For example, telethons may depict people with disabilities as weak and in need of charity. The hero stereotype provides a more positive representation of disability, though this form of "inspiration porn" or portrayal of a "supercrip" has also been criticized. In particular, the hero or supercrip narrative can suggest that a disability is something to be overcome rather than a different way of being. It may also imply that people can overcome disability with willpower and determination, leading to unrealistic expectations. This stereotype is often discussed with reference to sporting competitions such as the Paralympics (see *Sport and the supercrip* section, this chapter).

The third common stereotype portrays people with disabilities as a threat to society, particularly in relation to violent behaviour. Though this is often discussed with reference to mental health, the threat stereotype also applies to physical disability (e.g. Captain Hook in *Peter Pan*). This particular stereotype often implies that the disability is a punishment for evil or bad behaviour and that people with a disability are angry about their condition. The fourth stereotype suggests that people with disabilities are unable to adjust to their situation and, to some extent, are "their own worst enemy". For example, a person may be shown as refusing to use their mobility aids or take prescribed medication. This type of representation implies that the cause of difficulties associated with disability is the inability (or unwillingness) to engage with support, and hence minimizes the importance of societal stigma and a lack of suitable accommodation.

People with disabilities are frequently represented as a burden either to their primary support network or to wider society. The emphasis is typically on family members, partners, or paid carers and the sacrifices made by them when supporting a person with disabilities. In this manner the media treats the person who is disabled as little more than a prop or plot device, whilst the wider societal accommodations that would support people with disabilities (e.g. workplace accommodations) are ignored. The final stereotype is an extension of the burden stereotype and suggests that people with disabilities are "better off dead". Euthanasia is often central to the storyline, with the person who is disabled frequently expected or encouraged to "do the right thing" by ending their life to allow their loved ones to move on without the apparent burden of care. The portrayal often fails to discuss rehabilitative care or adjustment to a new diagnosis and the rich fulfilled lives that people with a disability can lead.

Disability drag

As discussed, there is a lack of disability representation in the media. It is, therefore, important that when people with disabilities are included, they are portrayed in an authentic and respectful manner. Even when characters with disabilities are sensitively created and portrayed, however, they often lack authenticity, as relatively few characters with disabilities are played by actors who themselves have that disability. For example, whilst Daniel Day-Lewis delivers an exceptional performance as writer and artist Christy Brown in *My Left Foot*, Day-Lewis does not himself have cerebral palsy.

This "disability drag" (i.e. the use of actors without a disability to play characters that have a disability) has been criticized by both disability activists and media commentators. Disability drag has also been compared to blackface and yellowface (i.e. the use of cosmetics by Caucasian actors to imitate characters from racial and ethnic minorities). As stated by Woodburn and Ruderman (2016), "Imagine if 95% of black characters were played by white actors. We as a society have accepted people's right to self-representation, and yet when it comes to people with disabilities, we're apparently fine with so-called cripface or disability drag."

In response to such criticism, it is often argued that casting non-disabled actors in these roles allows the media to show characters both before and after the disability develops. For example, films such as *You're Not You* (amyotrophic lateral sclerosis, ALS), *Still Alice* (Alzheimer's), and *The Theory of Everything* (ALS) illustrate the process of becoming disabled and adapting to disability. In one particularly prominent example, *Born on the Fourth of July*, there is a clear contrast between the young naïve Ron Kovic who enlists for service in Vietnam and the mature, determined man who becomes a leading disability activist.

Depicting characters both before and after onset of a disability may also remind audiences that anyone can become disabled and those without disabilities are *currently* or *temporarily* without disability – a distinction which may help reduce the stigma of disability. However, the casting of non-disabled actors to portray disabled characters often appears driven by the opportunity for non-disabled actors to excel (and therefore enhance the prestige of the film). Actors who portray disabled characters often receive critical praise with numerous performers receiving academy awards for their roles, including Jamie Foxx (*Ray*), Holly Hunter (*The Piano*), and Dustin Hoffman (*Rain Man*). Casting non-disabled actors in these roles does not, however, support the talented actors who are themselves disabled and can therefore provide a more authentic representation of disability.

Advertising

One sector of the media less likely to recruit non-disabled actors to represent disability (i.e. "disability drag") is advertising. In part, this may reflect false advertising legislation which prevents media "faking disability" and thus encourages advertising companies to hire actors and models who are themselves disabled. Organizations may also fear offending their disabled customers and a subsequent backlash against the product that they are trying to promote. Whether motivated by profit or social conscience, advertisements featuring people with disabilities have become more prominent (Haller & Ralph, 2001, 2006). Importantly, such representation appears to have moved from themes of dependency and pity to a more inclusive and empowering message.

Advertisements for aspirational products where the consumer is expected to desire to look or behave like the featured model (e.g. beauty products) are, however, less likely to feature disability. Indeed, where disability is featured the signs of visible difference are often minimized. For example, a model or actor is featured who uses a wheelchair but whose appearance and speech display no other signs of impairment. In one notable exception, the Cingular

Wireless advertisement featured an artist, Dan Keplinger, with cerebral palsy. The advertisement specifically focuses on ability and empowerment rather than charity and pity.

Similar to traditional product-based advertising, disability-focused charities also depict disabilities in order to generate donations. Traditionally, charities have often relied on images intended to elicit sympathy and pity. These may, however, reinforce the stereotyped notion that disabled people are dependent and in need of financial support and more recent images are less likely to adopt this approach. Relatively few studies have, however, considered the impact of such advertising. In one exception, Kamenetsky et al. (2016) presented undergraduate students with older (1960–1990) and more recent (1991–2010) disability charity images. Newer images led to more positive responses and there was no significant difference in the participants' willingness to help when viewing the older and more recent images. Findings suggest that willingness to help is not dependent on the use of images which elicit pity. Hence, more positive and empowering images should be adopted.

Mental health

Media representation of mental health is problematic. The prevalence of television characters depicting mental health conditions has increased in recent years (see Mantilla & Goggin, 2020 for details of representation in one popular drama). However, negative stereotypes persist, and whilst representation has generally improved, the media often miss important opportunities to challenge stereotypes and dispel common myths. Poor representation is not, of course, restricted to fictional dramas but instead occurs across a range of different media types. For example, negative references to mental health and mental health treatment are also found in children's television (Wahl, 2003). Lawson and Fouts (2004) report that 85% of Disney films contain some reference to mental health and the language adopted (e.g. "crazy" or "nuts") is typically used to derogate others or create fear. For example, in *Beauty and the Beast* one character makes reference to a "lunacy wagon".

Characters with mental health conditions are frequently depicted as violent, unpredictable, and a danger to society (Chen & Lawrie, 2017; Stuart, 2006). Such negative stereotypes appear to be a feature of both fictional and fact-based media, with sensationalist accounts more likely to capture the audience's attention, thus increasing ratings or publication figures. Mental health is also often linked to social isolation in the media, with characters who have mental health conditions frequently depicted without an occupation and distanced from their family or wider social network. Schizophrenia and conditions where no specific diagnosis is provided appear to receive the poorest treatment in the popular media (Pirkis & Francis, 2012).

Media representations of mental health can impact on prejudice and discrimination against those with mental health conditions. For example, in one study viewers of the movie *Joker* displayed higher levels of mental health-based prejudice than those watching an alternative movie (Scarf et al., 2020).

Further, Diefenbach and West (2007) report that television viewing is associated with the belief that placing mental health services in residential neighbourhoods endangers community members. These representation issues have widespread consequences. For example, media linking mental health with violent or risky behaviour can influence public debate, which influences subsequent policy and mental health practice (Hallam, 2002). Media portrayals may also impact on the wellbeing of individuals who themselves have mental health conditions, including the interpretation of symptoms and willingness to engage in treatment. For example, those who are more able to recall news stories involving violent or criminal acts performed by someone with a mental health condition are more reluctant to reveal a mental health condition themselves (Morgan & Jorm, 2009).

The media also has the potential to improve societal understanding of mental health and promote inclusion. In the Time to Change report, *Making a Drama out of a Crisis* (2014), 54% of respondents believed that television drama improved their understanding of mental health issues and 31% said that the television drama helped them to discuss mental health with family, friends, or colleagues. In addition, 25% of those experiencing a mental health issue were encouraged to seek professional help after viewing a character with a similar issue and 25% of those who knew someone with a mental health condition were prompted to make contact after viewing a television mental health storyline. Representation in television drama may be particularly impactful when the viewers have developed a relationship with the character over many years.

Relatively few studies have considered the potential for mass media interventions to reduce mental health-oriented prejudice and discrimination and additional research in this area is required (Clement et al., 2013). There is, however, some indication that documentary films, mass media stigma reduction campaigns, and online mental health literacy programmes may have a positive effect on the general public, particularly if these include the personal stories of people with mental health conditions (Pirkis & Francis, 2012). In addition, viewers often engage with mental health storylines beyond the onscreen episodes (e.g. discussing the issue on Facebook or Twitter) and there is considerable scope to strengthen this aspect of media coverage.

Disability-focused media and social media

One area of the media that has received little public recognition or systematic research attention is the media created by those who are themselves disabled. Example publications include *Able* magazine, *PosAbility* magazine, and *Disability Horizons* magazine. Though the internet has increased opportunities for such publications, disability-focused media are not a new phenomenon. Indeed, publications targeted at readers with disabilities and their support networks (i.e. families and friends of people with disabilities or the professionals who support them) have been produced for over a hundred years.

Disability-focused media were created, in part, as a response to the poor representation and stereotyping that exist in the mainstream media. Like other forms of alternative or minority publication that represent those who have been stigmatized or discriminated against, disability-focused media typically advocate on behalf of their community and draw attention to those issues that are neglected by the mainstream media. As stated by Gwin, the editor of one such publication (*Mouth*), "Nobody [in the non-disabled media] is going to cover the disability-rights movement, so we're just going to have to cover it our own damn selves" (Lathrop, 1995, p. 37). These publications may also have greater awareness of the need to provide media content in alternative formats such as audio or braille, or a greater willingness to do so.

Online media (e.g. Facebook, Twitter, Second Life, YouTube, blogs) also provide important opportunities for the disabled community to connect with others, obtain or disseminate information, coordinate activism, and challenge mainstream media narratives. Hence, whilst social media is often discussed with reference to the negative consequences of online engagement (e.g. Kelly et al., 2018), there are a number of advantages to online activity. Facebook is, of course, the most widely researched form of social networking, though disability-specific social networking sites (e.g. Disaboom.com, AbleHere.com, and ilivewithadisability.com) are also available. Indeed, it has been suggested that whilst people with disabilities use Facebook to connect to non-disabled friends and family, other platforms are favoured to engage with the disabled community (Shpigelman & Gill, 2014).

In one study analysing social media use, Caton and Chapman (2016) report that social media provides important opportunities for individuals with intellectual disabilities to express their social identity and to form or enhance personal relationships. Such opportunities may be particularly valuable for those based in rural communities or unable to travel to meet in person (Raghavendra et al., 2015). Indeed, people with disabilities are at greater risk of social isolation and loneliness. Many non-disabled people obtained more insight into the value of social media during the COVID-19 pandemic when physical distancing led to a reliance on online interaction. It is important that opportunities to interact online remain after the risk of contagion subsides.

Social media can be an important source of health information (e.g. Zhao & Zhang, 2017) and this may be particularly important for those seeking to understand or adjust to a new diagnosis or progression of their condition. Difficulties can arise, however, if the information is inaccurate or misleading (Bezin et al., 2017). Therefore, the accuracy and authenticity of the information disseminated is essential, particularly as misleading information may be more popular online than accurate public health information (Sharma et al., 2017). Though research has often focused on the dissemination of the "facts and figures", experiential information is also important. For example, YouTube and personal websites allow people with disabilities to provide a more personal insight into the lived experience of specific disabilities. Such posts may address both aspects of the condition (e.g. particular symptoms) and personal and social barriers to be addressed. Social media also provide a useful forum for instructional videos (Libin et al., 2011) and should, therefore, be further integrated into future healthcare provision (Naslund et al., 2016).

In many cases, social media content is created in order to challenge existing disability stereotypes, advocate for societal or policy change, and coordinate activism. Indeed, social media allows people with disabilities to bypass the traditional media who act as "gatekeepers" for media content in order to take greater control of the information available. As described by one blogger, William Peace (who blogs as Bad Cripple), "My experience with mainstream media has been overwhelmingly negative. The message the mainstream media wants to present is you're either a hero or a lazy shit and there is no in between" (quoted in Haller, 2010, p. 3). Social media enables users to raise awareness of issues that are not addressed by the mainstream press, for example to promote events and disseminate news. Twitter may be particularly advantageous with re-tweeting allowing topics to become widely distributed and capturing the attention of practitioners, policymakers, and journalists.

Language

Language has the power to frame the way that we think about ourselves, specific issues, and social or cultural groups (Entman, 2007). It is, therefore, important to consider the language that we adopt when talking about disability. For example, the phrases "confined to a wheelchair" and "wheelchair bound" (rather than "uses a wheelchair") emphasize the mobility aid rather than the person who is disabled and ignore the argument that it is the environment (e.g. a lack of wheelchair ramps) that is disabling rather than the physical condition. Similarly, these phrases fail to understand that for many with compromised mobility, mobility aids such as a wheelchair can be emancipatory and increase rather than decrease a person's engagement and activity. To an extent, the use of terms indicative of loss or tragedy may reflect the fears of those who are not disabled (i.e. fear of losing mobility) rather than the self-identity of people with disabilities.

Language that is widely used and accepted is often problematic. The activist Bill Bolt (in *Ragged Edge*, formerly *The Disability Rag*) summarizes the issues associated with the term "disabled": "If we are 'disabled', that is, 'without abilities' then what is this demand for equal employment, journalists likely think. On the other hand if we can work with only minimal special arrangements, then why do we need all kinds of government funds to live on?" (quoted in Haller, 2010, p. 53).

Reflecting the importance of language and the potential for the media to create, exacerbate, or challenge stereotypes, a number of guidelines have been created for media professionals. These include the Disability Language Style Guide (2018) created by the National Center on Disability and Journalism at Arizona State University. Recommendations include referring to a disability only when it is relevant to the story and adopting people-first rather than disability-first language. Of course, others may resist this type of good practice, which has sometimes been dismissed as "political correctness" or even worse as "political correctness gone mad" (Lea, 2010). It is also important to recognize that issues do not arise only when talking about people with disabilities. For example, the metaphoric use of terms such as "lame" or "blind" to refer to deficiency or weakness is also problematic.

Models of disability

Models can frame our understanding of disability (Llewellyn & Hogan, 2000). In this section, I describe the dominant models of disability (i.e. the medical and social models) before presenting two more recently discussed models. Presenting these models is not intended to suggest that these are the only available models of disability or that one model represents "good" or "bad" practice. Instead, they are used to illustrate the models that have influenced perceptions of disability and associated policy and practice. It is also important to note that although the social model is most widely accepted by the disabled community, many researchers argue that a single model cannot provide a complete explanation of disability (Pfeiffer, 2001), with each model more accurately perceived as raising important issues or providing a specific insight in a particular context or case.

The medical model

The medical model frames disability as a consequence of physiological damage caused by injury or disease. Disabled people are believed to be "in need" of treatment to restore "normal" bodily function. Therefore, whilst no attempts are made to change the social or cultural context in which disabled people live, the individual is required to physically transform to better "fit" their environment. Indeed, the medical model can be seen to pressure disabled people to fit into narrow definitions of normality in order to gain social acceptance. Both functional and aesthetic aspects of "normality" are perceived to be important, and the medical model is often associated with the use of prostheses such as artificial limbs. The medical model may, therefore, contribute to negative societal perceptions of disability by focusing on deficits and expecting disabled individuals to adopt a passive and secondary status.

Treatment and rehabilitation occur under the care and supervision of "expert" medical practitioners who are typically regarded as having a more informed understanding of the impairment than the disabled individual. Practitioners have considerable power and authority. Through diagnosis of a specific condition, they provide disabled people with access (or deny their access) to a range of services, accommodations, and benefits. Medical professionals adopt, therefore, the role of gatekeeper whilst disabled people become dependent on their decisions. Though practitioners are typically presented as caring and informed professionals, historical events such as the extermination and sterilization programmes implemented by the Nazi regime have been highlighted to provide a contrast to this compassionate image. As described by Gallager (1990), "The people who set up the euthanasia program were not madmen; nor were they, at least at the start, killers. They were doctors and bureaucrats, efficient men ... They sought to regularise and rationalise the disorderly state of nature: the life process is so often untidy and inefficient" (p. 56).

The medical model typically frames disability as an individual weakness and discussions of disability often focus on personal characteristics that facilitate recovery, such as a person's willpower and determination to "fight" their condition. Therefore, those who do not recover may be portrayed as lacking the "strength of character" required to overcome the condition. Indeed, those who do not wish to be "fixed" may be perceived as non-compliant or unmotivated (Roush & Sharby, 2011). Together with the concepts of "abnormality" and "deviation", this "unwillingness to recover" is one potentially stigmatizing aspect of the medical model. Brisenden (1986) provides a powerful critique of the medical model, arguing that although medical "facts" are useful, we require more than these to understand the lived experience of disability. According to Brisenden (1986), "we need to build up a picture of what it is like to be a disabled person in a world run by non-disabled people. This involves treating the experiences and opinions of people with disabilities as valid and important" (p. 173).

The social model

The social model distinguishes between impairment and disability. Impairment describes the (physical, mental, or sensory) function or dysfunction experienced, whilst disability is imposed by society and acts as a form of oppression. For example, people using a wheelchair may be impaired by a physical injury or illness, but it is the lack of wheelchair access in society that is disabling. As stated by Oliver (1996), "it is not individual limitations, of whatever kind, which are the cause of the problem but society's failure to provide appropriate services and adequately ensure [that] the needs of disabled people are fully taken into account in its social organization" (p. 32). Therefore, in placing the emphasis on society rather than the individual, the social model encourages disabled people to focus on transforming society rather than medical intervention.

Indeed, the social model has encouraged social and political activism that has improved the lives of many disabled people. It has promoted sustained and coordinated positive social change (e.g. campaigns for anti-discrimination legislation) and has encouraged a more emancipatory and inclusive approach to disability research. The model is one of the most prominent and influential narratives of the disability movement. Indeed, it has received wider (though not universal) acceptance amongst the disability community compared to the medical model. It is important to acknowledge that there are a number of versions of the social model, including the impairment, independent living, and postmodern versions, though they share core features (Mitra, 2006). Specifically, impairment is viewed as a biological state (e.g. restricted function) and disability is a consequence of societal structures that do not accommodate those impairments. Hence, disability is conceptualized as in addition to the initial biological impairment, and social isolation and exclusion represent important themes. In this manner, it is society rather than the individual that is targeted for intervention.

For some critics, the social model neglects the impact of the condition itself on the individual. Supporters of the social model have claimed that "Once social barriers to the reintegration of people with physical impairments are removed, the disability itself is eliminated. The requirements are for changes to society, material changes to the environment, changes in environmental control systems, changes in social roles, and changes in attitudes" (Finkelstein, 1980, p. 33). However, as a disabled person myself this does not fully capture my experience and acknowledging biological aspects of the impairment (e.g. chronic pain) does not reduce the importance I place on discrimination or structural inequalities. As summarized by Crow (1996), "for many disabled people personal struggles relating to impairment will remain even when disabling barriers no longer exist" (p. 209).

Shakespeare and Watson (2001) also highlight the role of biological impairment for many supporters of the social model, stating: "Most activists concede that behind closed doors they talk about aches and pains and urinary tract infections, even while they deny any relevance of the body while they are out campaigning, yet this inconsistency is surely wrong" (p. 12). In response, advocates of the model argue that they do not deny the impact of physical impairment but that this is distinct from disability. Additional criticisms are that the social model neglects the importance of intersectionality (e.g. race and ethnicity) and differences between individuals with the same physical symptoms and prognosis.

Alternative models

Although the medical and social models of disability have dominated discussions, alternative models of disability have been proposed, including the capability model (Sen, 1985) and affirmation model (Swain & French, 2000). These are not necessarily intended to replace the medical or social model, as one overarching model of disability may be unrealistic. Instead, they highlight issues that have been neglected by previous models and different ways to conceptualize disability. The capability model (Sen, 1985) considers the economic causes and consequences of disability, focusing on an individual's capability to function (i.e. what they are able to do) rather than their income. Disability is conceptualized as compromised capability (i.e. opportunities) or functioning (i.e. achievement), which is a consequence of personal characteristics (e.g. gender, the specific impairment), the resources available (e.g. income), the environment (e.g. socio-political and cultural), or the interaction between these.

For example, energy-limiting conditions may be disabling regardless of resources. However, those with financial resources may be able to reduce the impact of disability by paying for childcare or a cleaner to support household tasks. Indeed, in many countries the resources available to a person may also determine their access to diagnostic tests, prescribed drugs, or medical care. In this manner, different individual experiences of the same condition (dependent on the context and individual affected) are recognized. A distinction is also made between potential disability (affecting an individual's opportunities) and actual disability (impacting on their achievement). Therefore, the capability model provides valuable context for the person's lived experience. Other models may question whether an individual is capable of walking a specific distance (i.e. the medical model), as required for some benefit claims, or if social structures create additional barriers to those not capable of doing so (i.e. the social model) without considering the extent to which they wish to do so as part of their daily life. Of course, the capability model cannot easily categorize individuals as disabled or not disabled (a core focus of the medical model) as is typically required for individuals to receive accommodations or external support.

Models of disability often adopt a deficit-based approach, focusing on what a person cannot do in a narrative that focuses on personal tragedy and loss. For example, accounts may state that "a young woman with her whole life ahead of her was struck down (by illness or accident) leaving her unable to walk, hear, etc.". The affirmation model is a response to such personal tragedy narratives and places greater emphasis on disabled people living rich and fulfilling lives. Swain and French (2000) describe the model of disability as offering "a non-tragic view of disability and impairment which encompasses positive social identities, both individual and collective, for disabled people grounded in the benefits of lifestyle and life experience of being impaired and disabled" (p. 569). Indeed, many disabled people highlight the strengths or opportunities afforded by disability, such as greater empathy and the richness of disability culture.

Conducting research: nothing about us without us

People with disabilities are often marginalized, with professionals or family members making decisions about the rights and treatment of the person who is disabled rather than the person who is disabled making decisions for themselves. A similar trend occurs on a larger scale, such as the design and implementation of national policy. Those without disabilities may have less insight into the experience of disability, but as professionals they may be regarded as an "expert" on the condition, with their recommendations having a substantial impact on practice. The statement "nothing about us without us" has been employed by disability rights activists to campaign that policy decisions should require full participation by stakeholder representatives. The principle also applies to research and wider care or treatment issues.

For academic medical conferences, Chu et al. (2016) propose four principles of patient involvement for conference organizers: (1) accommodation;

(2) co-design; (3) engagement; and (4) education and mentorship. Accommodation refers to the venue, travel, and hotel arrangements. For example, conferences increasingly provide "quiet rooms" for delegates who may need to rest, or online streaming of the conference for those unable to attend in person. Patient representation is often tokenistic and the co-design principle requires that patient representatives and conference organizers are afforded equal status and involvement. For example, patients should be provided with the same opportunities to identify overarching conference themes and select speakers. Engagement refers to patient involvement in the conference as both speakers and attendees, with no sessions closed to patients or their representatives. Conferences should also provide patients with opportunities to learn how to engage with researchers and other relevant parties (education and mentorship).

Although meaningful engagement by people with disabilities strengthens each stage of the research process, it is important to recognize that participation in research may be emotionally and physically demanding. For example, participants who are comfortable in the researcher's presence may feel able to discuss topics that they did not anticipate disclosing (Vaughan et al., 2019), which may contribute to feelings of vulnerability or unease. Of course, discussing sensitive issues (such as disability or stigma) may also impact on the researcher and it is important that all those engaged in this area are prepared for such eventualities.

Studies conducted by academics who are themselves disabled are not necessarily without difficulties. For example, although disability may increase awareness of issues such as stigma or navigating workplace accommodations, researchers may investigate conditions other than their own and having one condition does not provide an understanding of another disability. Even when an academic examines their own condition, difficulties may arise. Sharing one identity (e.g. blind) with a participant does not mean that the researcher and participant have other shared experiences and understandings (e.g. gender, ethnicity, sexuality, socio-economic status). The shared identity of a specific condition may provide a false confidence that the researcher can understand the participant's perspective, leading to assumptions and misunderstandings. Indeed, experiences of the same condition vary with regards to the severity and frequency of symptoms, availability of support, and acceptance of the condition, giving rise to very different personal experiences.

Summary

A number of issues should be considered to contextualize the experience of disabled academics. First, representations of disability are commonly negative, portraying disabled people as a threat, burden, or source of pity. Such representations contribute to an environment that is hostile to individuals with disabilities. Second, dominant models of disability frame disability in markedly different ways, with important implications for disability-related practice and policy. It is important to consider such approaches to disability, which may, for example, influence attitudes towards engagement with the medical profession and disability activism. Finally, the voices of disabled people have often been silenced in favour of non-disabled medical experts. This has occurred both in relation to their own impairment and wider disability issues. Those conducting research in this area should adopt a more collaborative approach, conducting research *with* disabled people rather than *on* disabled people. Their voices are important and deserve to be heard.

Sport and the supercrip stereotype

DePauw (1997) identifies three stages of disability representation in sport. People with disabilities are: (1) invisible or excluded from sport (i.e. invisibility of disability in sport); (2) visible in sport as disabled athletes (i.e. visibility of disability in sport); or (3) are becoming visible in sport as athletes (i.e. (in) visibility of disability in sport). Depending on the nature of the sport, people with disabilities arguably remain in the first or second stage, i.e. excluded from sport or recognized as disabled athletes. In contrast, the final stage, whereby people with disabilities are visible primarily as athletes, remains relatively rare. For example, DePauw cites the example of winter ski competitions which rank athletes with and without disabilities alongside each other.

Both the Olympic and Paralympic Games attract a considerable media audience. Coverage includes the sporting events themselves and a range of associated activities such as the opening and closing ceremonies, athlete profiles, and product endorsements. In recent years, the profile of the Paralympic Games has increased with important opportunities to challenge existing disability-related stereotypes. Indeed, a central aspect of the 2012 London Paralympic Games was to promote disability rights and improve long-term opportunities for disabled people. However, media coverage remains problematic, and it has been suggested that there is a hierarchy of disability with, for example, athletes who use wheelchairs more likely to be featured in the media than athletes with cerebral palsy (Schell & Duncan, 1999).

When disabled people compete in sporting events, the hero or supercrip stereotype is common, which suggests that the individual should be celebrated for "overcoming" their disability and achieving sporting success despite this disadvantage. Silva and Howe (2012) provide a critique of the supercrip Paralympic narrative. Though the supercrip narrative may appear to empower people with disabilities, Silva and Howe argue that it reflects the low social expectations of those with disabilities where any achievement (e.g. athletic or career success) is elevated and perceived as surprising. It also reflects the othering of people with disabilities who are framed as different from "normal" athletes. Hence, it has been argued that the frequent use of personal interest stories frames the Paralympic Games as a "spectacle" rather than a sporting event.

Indeed, the extent to which disabled athletes are presented as elite sports men and women rather than objects of interest could be questioned. The Paralympic Games receive less extensive coverage than the Olympic Games and athletes with disabilities are less likely than their non-disabled peers to be featured in the media outside the context of the Games. Further, in one content analysis of the 2016 Olympic and Paralympic Games, Rees et al. (2019) argue that the Paralympic Games is framed as an entertainment show rather than a sporting event, with more frequent attempts to elicit emotion in the Paralympic Games and a greater emphasis on participation than competition. For instance, Beacom et al. (2016) highlight the prominence of tragedy and transformation narratives around the 2012 London and 2014 Sochi Paralympic Games, in which overcoming a disability and the nature of the disability itself are framed first rather than the athlete. Such coverage may signal that the Paralympics are a less serious competition than the Olympic Games and that those competing at the Paralympics are not "real" athletes.

Teachers and academics in the media

The media has the potential to educate the general population about professional roles and associated policy issues, including the role of academics and issues impacting on the education sector. Movies highlighting social injustice and educational reform may be particularly beneficial (Raimo et al., 2002). Compared with other professions (e.g. lawyers, medical practitioners), however, educators featured in the media spend relatively little time practising their occupation (Heilman, 1991). As a consequence, the media provides the audience with little understanding of the role and responsibilities of teachers and academics. Indeed, those who are inspired to become teachers by these popular media portrayals may have a distorted expectation of the teacher role (e.g. the workload) and be relatively unprepared for their position. Similarly, the media may encourage students and parents to develop unrealistic expectations of the student–teacher relationship (Swetnam, 1992).

There are a number of media stereotypes associated with the teaching profession. In one analysis of American films (1939–2003) featuring teachers, Beyerbach (2005) identifies three common themes: "Fast Times", "Dangerous Minds", and "Stand on Me". The "Fast Times" theme focuses on students as increasingly uncontrollable and immoral, regardless of the period in which the movie is set or released. In these movies, educators often focus on "saving" their students from the social and moral threats they encounter. "Dangerous Minds" highlights the potential for education (and therefore educators and students) to challenge and reform the system, whilst the "Stand on Me" theme portrays teachers as powerless against the tradition and bureaucracy that is pervasive in society and education more specifically.

One further common form of representation is the "superhuman" teacher. As depicted in the movies *Dangerous Minds* and *Freedom Writers*, these teachers are able to support their students on both a personal and professional (i.e. academic) level where others have repeatedly failed (or failed to care). Whilst highlighting the transformative nature of education, this stereotyped image sets an unrealistic standard for teachers. As stated by Raphael (1985), "Teachers who internalize these unrealistic expectations are being set up for disappointment. They start making demands upon themselves which they cannot possibly achieve. Unsuccessful, they become frustrated and they tend to blame themselves for failing to attain impossible goals" (p. 9).

The "superhuman teachers" are typically depicted as relentlessly positive, with unlimited energy to invest in their students' personal lives. There are, therefore, important parallels with the "supercrip" narrative where people with disabilities "overcome" their condition, almost by willpower and strength of character alone. The depiction of a "superhuman" teacher fails to acknowledge the excessive workloads experienced by many educators or the importance of maintaining educator wellbeing. The "superhuman" teacher characters are often featured in direct contrast to (typically older and more experienced) teachers or administrative staff who adhere more strictly to the rules and regulations of their organization. In this manner, those who do not make such personal sacrifices ("superhuman" teachers often risk their jobs to support their students) are portrayed as selfish, bitter, and uncaring. Indeed, an important aspect of the "superhuman" narrative is that teachers must be unconventional and challenge authority in order to be successful.

Movies centred on higher education rather than secondary education also feature such stereotypes. For example, in *Mona Lisa Smile* the central character challenges existing social conventions and specifically the expectation that female students should aspire to marry and raise children rather than enter a career. Many movies based in a university setting focus on extra-curricular activities and the lives of the students with only peripheral academic roles (e.g. *The Social Network*). Educators with a disability are also rarely featured in the mass media, though disabled students (receiving the care of a non-disabled teacher) are more common (Beyerbach, 2005). Prominent media representation of academics with disabilities or long-term health conditions include *Still Alice* (Alzheimer's). Here the academic role is presented as an illustration of the capable and confident professional role that cannot be maintained when the dementia advances. There is, therefore, a lack of disabled role models for teachers and academics or those considering such a career.

2 Stigma and discrimination

Research demonstrates that people with visible or known disabilities continue to experience a range of prejudice and discrimination in society. This extends to the workplace with disability-related prejudice and discrimination evident at each stage of the recruitment, employment, and progression process. People may engage in a process of "covering" in which they attempt to hide the stigma-causing attribute (e.g. disability) and deflect attention away from it. However, those attempting to "pass" as non-disabled may experience considerable distress when trying to conceal symptoms and may not receive access to valuable support (e.g. visible walking aids). Chapter 2 considers the experience of stigma and discrimination and the consequences of this for disabled academics.

Defining stigma

Martin (2010) describes stigma as "a socially constructed mark of disapproval, shame, or disgrace that causes significant disadvantage through the curtailment of opportunities" (p. 261). According to Goffman (1963), stigma reduces its bearer "from a whole and usual person to a tainted and discounted one" (p. 3). He identifies three categories of stigma: "tribal identity" (e.g. race and ethnicity), "abominations of the body" (e.g. physical abnormalities), and "blemishes of character" (e.g. mental illness). Goffman (1963) also distinguishes between discredited and discreditable attributes. Discredited attributes refer to obvious and visible signs of "deviance" such as a wheelchair or walking aid, whereas discreditable attributes are differences that may impact on the individual's reputation but are not immediately apparent to observers.

For people with disabilities that are clearly visible (or known) to others, stigma can impact on the way in which they are perceived and treated by others. For example, stigma has an important impact on employer compliance with discrimination legislation (Scheid, 2005). Those with discreditable attributes (such as invisible health conditions) are typically assumed to be "normal" (i.e. healthy) and must decide whether to disclose their stigmatized identity or not. As Goffman (1963) states, "To display or not to display; to tell or not to tell; to let on or not to let on; to lie or not to lie; and in each case, to whom, how, when, and where" (p. 42). Those wishing to conceal a discreditable attribute may ascribe behaviour associated with that attribute to a non-stigmatizing condition or behaviour. For example, tiredness could be attributed to a lack of sleep rather than a medical impairment. As described by one of the disabled academics I interviewed,

> "If I miss something, because I can't get in, I usually say I'm having an asthma attack. I don't say I haven't got the energy to come into work. I just lie. Because I do have asthma. You know, I just say, 'I've been up all night, I couldn't breathe. I'm really tired'" (Academic 5).

Alternatively, individuals may be selective about who they do or do not disclose to (see Chapter 4 for a more detailed discussion of these issues).

Though the subject of stigma is most commonly associated with Goffman (1963), other theorists have further developed this concept or proposed alternative categories and classification of stigma types. Jones and Corrigan (2014) propose four types of stigma: public stigma (i.e. widespread stereotypes about disability and specific conditions), self-stigma (i.e. internalization of a stereotype and application of this stereotype to the self), label avoidance (e.g. refusal to access services to avoid being categorized as disabled or stereotyped), and structural stigma (i.e. intentional and unintentional regulations that discriminate against individuals). Public and structural stigma are, perhaps, the most commonly recognized or discussed forms of stigma. For example, these are often the focus of research, activism, and subsequent policy. It is important to acknowledge, however, that self-stigma and label avoidance also impact on the wellbeing of disabled people.

For example, disabled people who accept negative stereotypes about disability or their specific condition (e.g. that disabled people are less capable, experienced, or important than those without disabilities) may withdraw from social interaction, become isolated, attempt to conceal their condition, and reject treatment and support (Jennings et al., 2015; Oliveira et al., 2015). Self-stigma and label avoidance impact on the experiences of disabled academics. For example, Academic 4 described distancing herself from the term disabled: "*I do count myself as somebody who has a disability, but I won't ... It's not a label that I attach to myself publicly very often because of the stigma around it.*"

Academic 4 explained the impact of self-stigma on their engagement with support services: "*I did involve the Union, the second time I was signed off. So I have a caseworker. And he came to my meetings, when I was going back on phased return and stuff. And that was good, because I didn't involve them the first time around. Because I just felt like ... because of just the, I guess my own internalized ableism actually was like, 'I don't need that support' ... So I had to confront a lot of stuff about myself, actually, and my own judgements of disability and kind of stuff like that, and what that meant to me, and that was quite weird, going through that process. But I'm glad I did. Obviously.*"

Indeed, developing and maintaining a positive self-identity may be difficult for stigmatized individuals who "... have (or are believed to have) an attribute that marks them as different and leads them to be devalued in the eyes of others" (Major & O'Brien, 2005, p. 395). Self-stigma involves an awareness of widespread stereotypes, agreement with those stereotypes, and application of the stereotype to the self. In one account, Battye (1966) states:

"Somewhere deep inside us is the almost unbearable knowledge that the way the able-bodied world regards us is as much as we have the right to expect. We are not full members of that world, and the vast majority of us can never hope to be" (pp. 8–9). This may, to some extent, explain why many people who meet formal disability criteria do not identify as disabled or seek the accommodations available (Grewal et al., 2002). Wider societal ramifications of self-stigma and label avoidance also exist. For example, reluctance to identify as disabled may impede the organization and effectiveness of disabled activism (Watson, 2002).

Stigma and disability

The extent to which specific conditions are stigmatized and the impact of this stigma on an individual varies widely. Jones et al. (1984) identified six specific dimensions of stigma that may influence the extent to which particular conditions are stigmatized. These dimensions are concealability, course, disruptiveness, aesthetic qualities, origin, and peril. *Concealability* refers to the visibility of the condition and the extent to which that visibility is controllable. It is important to note that visibility may not be stable and the visibility of an impairment may vary over time or in different contexts. For example, a condition may be more visible when a person interacts with others or when mobile. *Course* relates to the degree of change in the condition over time and the *disruptiveness* is the impact of the condition on the individual, for example the extent to which it may impact on interpersonal relationships.

Aesthetic qualities refer to the change to a person's appearance and the extent to which the stigmatizing condition may make an individual less "appealing" or more upsetting to others. This may of course extend beyond the direct effects of the condition. For example, weight gain as an indirect result of a mobility issue or fatigue may also be stigmatized. The *origin* dimension relates to the source of the condition. In particular, conditions perceived to have developed as a consequence of an individual's "risky" behaviour are often more stigmatized than where there is believed to be no personal responsibility. We may, of course, further differentiate between the apparent responsibility for developing the stigmatizing condition and for maintaining it. Finally, *peril* constitutes the threat posed by the condition and stigmatized individual. For example, people with mental health conditions may be stereotyped as unpredictable or dangerous, whilst other conditions may appear to present a risk of contagion (see Chapter 1 for a discussion of common disability stereotypes).

As discussed in the next section, considerable attention (in both research and practice) has been paid to the different levels of stigma associated with individual conditions. It is important, however, to acknowledge that the same conditions or cues may be perceived differently depending on the individual presenting with the condition or symptom or the context in which it occurs. For example, women who use wheelchairs may be more stigmatized than male wheelchair users. It has been argued that whilst men who use wheelchairs are presumed to be disabled through injury (e.g. military service or motorbike injury), female wheelchair users are believed to have a medical condition prompting perceptions of vulnerability or fear of contagion.

Female academics with disabilities may be especially disadvantaged. Indeed, the bias and discrimination experienced by female academics (regardless of their disability status) is well documented (e.g. Files et al., 2017; Krawczyk & Smyk, 2016; MacNell et al., 2015). As summarized by one academic: *"They're gonna be looking down a) on females and doubly so on disabled people, because they would, I would think, conceive of it as a deficit. You know, that they're not really good enough, they're the also rans, and that kind of thing, you know"* (Academic 10). Similarly, another academic commented: *"I think female academics already have to do more than males to succeed in academia. And I think they, if they see any weakness, then I don't think it's necessarily consciously, but they see that as a reflection of your ability"* (Academic 5).

Indeed, there are parallels between disability and other protected characteristics. Describing her experience, Academic 11 stated: *"It feels very similar, in some ways, to being female in academia, to being queer in academia. It's just, and I'm sure although I don't experience it, I'm sure being brown in academia is very similar as well. It's this, because you are not fitting in the majority path, they're not quite sure what to do with you. And if you work really hard to carve out your own little special place, maybe they'll let you stay there. But I can't see how you do that. There's not a path to it. That's the whole point. There's not a path to it."*

Conditions susceptible to stigma

Some impairments are particularly susceptible to misconceptions and stigma. These include those conditions that are misattributed to "inappropriate" behaviour such as sexual activity or smoking. This stigma has important ramifications for attitudes and behaviour towards those with the condition and for wider policy and practice, such as funding decisions. For example, lung cancer may receive less attention and research funding than other cancers because the condition is associated with smoking. Indeed, lung cancer patients often report feeling blamed for their condition even when they have never smoked or have not smoked for a number of years and this stigma negatively impacts on their quality of life (Brown Johnson et al., 2014; Chapple et al., 2004). This section considers the experience of two particularly stigmatized conditions: schizophrenia and HIV/AIDS.

Schizophrenia

Despite a number of high-profile education campaigns, the stigma associated with mental health persists. Research indicates that schizophrenia is one of the most stigmatized mental health conditions. Of particular concern, stigma is also evident among medical professionals (Llerena et al., 2002), which may impact on the level or type of support provided to service users. Stereotypes often associate schizophrenia with violence and unpredictability (Angermeyer & Schulze, 2001), promoting fear and avoidance of those with the condition. Such misconceptions are often perpetuated by the media and public education campaigns have had little impact on tackling these common stereotypes (Owen, 2012).

People with schizophrenia often anticipate that they will be viewed or treated unfavourably because of their condition and avoid disclosing their diagnosis (Lee et al., 2005). As described by one individual, "I don't tell members of the public. I mean people I don' know, not any more ... They think you're a f**king ... nutter" (Knight et al., 2003, p. 217). These concerns are not unfounded, with 55% and 43% of schizophrenia outpatients reporting that they had been exposed to offensive statements or media portrayals about people with psychiatric conditions respectively (Dickerson et al., 2002). It is, therefore, essential that negative representations in the media are actively challenged.

Stigma, both with respect to the stigma displayed by others and self-stigma reported by the service user, impacts on mental and physical wellbeing. For example, people with schizophrenia who are resistant to stigma demonstrate higher self-esteem, empowerment, and quality of life and lower levels of depression (Sibitz et al., 2011). In addition, those with higher levels of self-stigma are less likely to adhere to treatment programmes (Fung et al., 2008). Despite this, there has been little appreciation of the experience of academics with schizophrenia. Crompton (2017), however, reports that although the condition is stigmatized, being open about her own condition has allowed her to receive the support she needs. Saks also revealed her condition to colleagues, publishing a book entitled *The Center Cannot Hold* (2008) on her experience. Prior to this she disclosed to relatively few people, acknowledging: "I couldn't risk my illness being somehow exposed, certainly not before I'd achieved tenure" (p. 279).

HIV/AIDS

Whereas schizophrenia-related stereotypes are centred on violent and unpredictable behaviour, HIV/AIDS-related stigma is typically centred on fear of contagion and the behaviours historically associated with the condition (Rao et al., 2008). For people with HIV, these aspects of the stigma (i.e. contagion and blame) are particularly salient. As one person described it, "I really resent that there is an 'A' list and a 'B' list ... If I tell them that I got it from a transfusion, then I'm the victim, but if I got it from having sex then I have scarlet letters on my chest" (Sayles et al., 2007, p. 818). This stigma has a substantial impact on the experience of HIV/AIDS, physical health, and quality of life (Holzemer et al., 2009). For example, those experiencing stigma are less likely to adhere to a treatment regime (Rintamaki et al., 2006).

There has been little systematic research investigating the lived experience of academics with HIV/AIDS. Where research focused on higher education has been conducted, it has typically addressed the impact of education on student knowledge and understanding of HIV/AIDS, or the experiences of students with HIV/AIDS. In one anonymous account, an academic describes the stigma, isolation, and discrimination they experienced when disclosing their condition to colleagues or mentors (Anon., 2018). Hence, additional research and interventions are required. In particular, there has been little appreciation of advances in the treatment and management of the condition or the positive impact of employing faculty with such traditionally misunderstood conditions. For example, students receiving HIV/AIDS education display greater knowledge and more positive attitudes towards the condition when the academic reveals their HIV status (Scollay et al., 1992). This may be particularly important when there are relatively few opportunities for students to directly interact with those with specific conditions such as HIV/AIDS.

Workplace discrimination

There are two forms of stigma associated with discrimination: enacted stigma (i.e. actual incidence of discrimination) and felt stigma (i.e. fear of enacted discrimination) (Ragins, 2008). Though the majority of attention has focused on experience of actual enacted stigma, felt stigma needs also to be addressed. As described by one disabled employee, "I will always be under scrutiny because of what I represent – a disabled manager. I feel like I am on permanent probation in the sense that I feel the need to work super-hard to be on a par with my colleagues" (Roulestone & Williams, 2014, p. 25).

Felt stigma is also apparent within education. For example, dyslexic students report concerns that their thoughts and ideas are not clearly expressed and that others do not perceive them to be capable or intelligent, making many reluctant to contribute in group situations. As described by one student, "[J]ust be quiet, just be quiet and don't speak, because then [you won't] make an idiot out of yourself" (Cameron, 2016, p. 230). It is important, therefore, to acknowledge that negative attitudes towards disability create a hostile environment for disabled employees regardless of whether they have personally chosen to disclose a disability. As a consequence, many disabled students do not seek support due to fear of stigmatization and discrimination (Martin, 2010; Zaussinger & Terzieva, 2018).

With regards to enacted stigma, disabled people may be subject to both active (e.g. harassment, verbal abuse, physical violence) and passive (e.g. neglect, exclusion, removal of support) mistreatment. Disabled employees are subject to substantial workplace discrimination (Draper et al., 2011; McMahon & Shaw, 2005). For example, cross-culturally and across sectors, disabled people are less likely to be in paid employment (Sampson, 2003; Shah, 2005). In one experimental study, Ameri et al. (2018) sent job applications to over 6,000 employers. Applications either made no mention of disability or made a reference to a condition unlikely to impact on their performance (i.e. a spinal cord injury or Asperger's syndrome). Applications referencing disability received 26% fewer expressions of interest from employers. Some disabilities are, however, perceived to be more "acceptable" than others. In general, employers are more accepting of employees with physical or sensory impairments than an intellectual disability (Geng-quing & Qu, 2005). For example, in one study employers were more interested in hiring applicants with a physical disability, followed by those with ADHD; people with an acquired brain injury were perceived as the least desirable employees (Andersson et al., 2015).

Disabled people are, of course, aware of the stigma and discrimination targeted at people with disabilities. This presents particular challenges during the job application process. As explained by one person, "you just don't walk in and say, 'I am a manic depressive and a recovering alcoholic. How would you like to hire me?'" (Freedman & Fesko, 1996, p. 52). Similarly, one academic I interviewed described the difficulties associated with part-time work: "*One can, I understand, ask 'Would you consider part-time applications? Would you consider a job share? Would you ...', you know it's not completely unknown. But for one thing, that is an additional barrier that other people who can work full-time don't need to go through. It also means that I'm going to have to disclose in advance, probably, to somebody why I'm asking, why I want this job part-time. And that does prejudice people*" (Academic 12).

Previous research has placed greater emphasis on the exclusion of disabled people from the workplace than their experiences in paid employment. Disabled people are, however, also disadvantaged when employed. Disabled people are more likely than their non-disabled colleagues to be on part-time, temporary, or other forms of non-standard contract, typically with lower salaries and fewer benefits (Schur, 2003). Disability is also associated with lower job security, less training, fewer opportunities for decision-making, less institutional support, and more negative attitudes towards the organization and job (Schur et al., 2009; Wilson-Kovacs et al., 2008).

There are significant benefits for employers who hire, retain, and accommodate disabled employees (Hartnett et al., 2011). These benefits include retention of high-quality employees, increased employee productivity, and avoidance of costs required to recruit and train new members of staff. In addition, employees are aware that their value is recognized and appreciated, there is a more positive organizational culture, and the organization is more profitable (Hartnett et al., 2011). Despite this, discrimination against people with disabilities remains widespread. Indeed, even in occupations where disabled employees may provide important personal experience and understanding such as the health or caring professions, disabled employees report negative attitudes from their non-disabled colleagues (French, 1988). In particular, employers are often concerned that there is a financial cost associated with the employment of disabled workers – for example, to provide workplace accommodations (Kaye et al., 2011).

Workplace accommodations

Employers often express concern about the potential cost of workplace accommodations (i.e. adjustments to the role or work environment that are made to support the disabled employee). Despite this, there are a number of direct and indirect benefits associated with these accommodations. As noted previously, direct benefits include increased employee productivity, retention of qualified employees, and avoiding the cost of training new employees (Solovieva et al., 2011). Indirect benefits include improved quality of employee interactions, organizational morale, and organizational productivity (Solovieva et al., 2011).

Purchasing equipment and altering work schedules are among the most commonly reported accommodations. As Academic 11 explained, organizations may be more confident implementing these types of accommodation: "*I think people generally accept better the conditions where it's very clear-cut what people need. Where like, you know, all wheelchairs need ramps, it's a very nice simple rule and people can understand that. Whereas things like cognitive impairment, things like fatigue, you know, one person might need a space to nap, another person might just need like the understanding that sometimes they'll be moving a bit slower or need a shorter day.*"

To some extent, this may reflect a poor understanding of some impairments. Academic 11 recalled: "*I've asked for nap space at work. And one of the things they asked was 'oh, how long do you need to nap for instance [laughs], when will you need to do it [laughs]'. Like I can't, it's not a scheduled nap guys. I'm not like a toddler we're putting down after they've had their snack at lunch. It's sometimes I may be overcome with fatigue and need to lie down.*" Similarly, Academic 12 commented on her experience of a fluctuating condition: "*I don't know whether or not I'm going to need that accommodation every day. I don't know if I will need it this week. But I might suddenly need it on Wednesday next week. And if I don't have it, it's going to really, really cock my life up.*"

Disabled employees, however, be reluctant to request workplace accommodations (Baldridge & Veiga, 2001). This reluctance to request accommodations may reflect the negative attention and discrimination that is often directed at those receiving support. For example, service dogs support people with a range of impairments, including visual, auditory, neurological, and mental health conditions. Approximately half of service dog handlers report experiencing discrimination and those with disabilities that are not directly visible to others are particularly susceptible to discrimination (Mills, 2017). For example, over 75% of people with an invisible condition reported "often" experiencing invasive questioning in relation to their use of a service dog compared with 57% of those with a visible disability. Similarly, 82% of those with an invisible impairment reported that the legitimacy of their service dog use had been questioned, compared with 50% of those with a visible impairment. Therefore, using a service dog prevents people with invisible conditions from "passing" as non-disabled and exposes them to accusations of faking it or malingering. Such discrimination may discourage disabled people from accessing important sources of support (for more information on this, see Chapter 4).

Negative attention from colleagues may be especially hurtful. In one experimental study investigating employee disability, workplace accommodations, and perceived fairness, Paetzold et al. (2008) found that when a disabled employee excels at work, it is perceived by others as less fair than when they do not excel and is perceived to be least fair when a disabled employee both receives workplace accommodations and performs highly. In an educational context, the desire to avoid negative social reactions can deter disabled students from obtaining the necessary support (Lyman et al., 2016; Marshak et al., 2009). In particular, disabled students report concerns centred on the responses of their peers and tutors, fearing that they will be viewed as a burden, treated differently, or perceived to be seeking 'special' (advantageous) treatment that they did not deserve. One student reported, "They're like, labelling you and can't see you as an individual" (Prowse, 2009, p. 91). Hence, the fear of being stigmatized creates a barrier for those wishing to access disability services (Collins & Mowbray, 2005).

Perceived competence

Discrimination often relates to perceived competence or capability. This is often centred on the belief that disabled employees may not have the competence, ability, or experience required by the role, for example that they could not cope with a large workload or would be unreliable. One employer commented, "They wouldn't be able to either do the work efficiently or effectively; therefore, they would affect the bottom line" (Lengnick-Hall et al., 2008, p. 259). Similarly, another employer discussing disabled employees stated, "I have to be sure that if it is decided that you will begin at seven this week, that you don't come in at nine and say that you couldn't get up. That wouldn't work. It would be too hard for the rest of us who are working" (Strindlund et al., 2019, p. 2913).

In part this may reflect benevolent, paternalistic, or condescending ableism, where those without disability provide pity or unwanted help and infantilize those with disabilities (Nario-Redmond et al., 2019). Competence-related stereotypes not only exclude disabled people from the workplace, low expectations of disabled employees also reduce opportunities for people with disabilities to demonstrate their skills. As described by one disabled person, "You are not necessarily given the cutting-edge stuff, you're often given the safer pieces of work rather than the cutting edge so you're not stretching and therefore because you are not stretching you're not necessarily learning" (Wilson-Kovacs et al., 2008, p. 709).

Academia, stigma, and discrimination

Relatively few studies have considered the experiences of disabled academics. Indeed, academia often places greater emphasis on the diversity of their faculty with respect to other protected characteristics such as gender and ethnicity than disability (Steinberg et al., 2002). Research indicates, however, that similar to other professions, disabled people are less prevalent in academic roles than in the general population, particularly when a workplace accommodation is required (Mellifont et al., 2019). In one study focused on the experiences of 1,880 university employees, Snyder et al. (2010) demonstrate that disabled employees report more subtle and overt discrimination and more procedural injustice than their non-disabled colleagues. Disabled employees with non-physical disabilities are especially susceptible to such negative experiences.

One disabled academic commented, "It is like you are in a war; a war with yourself and with an ableist profession and environment that in so many ways constructs barriers to participation of disabled people" (Chouinard, 1995, p. 4). The academic environment often fails to accommodate or support disabled people, with respect to the physical space, the type of work conducted, and attitudes towards disability. Workspaces, including university buildings and campuses, are primarily designed for those without disabilities. Indeed, for historical buildings (that are often deemed to be the most prestigious), disabled access may only be permissible via retroactive accommodations and refurbishment. As a consequence, disabled academics and students constitute a minority, secondary concern.

As recalled by one of my interviewees: *"We had another lady who had physical disabilities and couldn't get upstairs. And when they timetabled in buildings where there was no lift, they said, 'Well, you'd have to just shuffle up on your bottom'. So they don't even look after people who have got obvious disabilities, never mind people who've got invisible disabilities"* (Academic 5). A lack of guidance and information is also apparent to disabled academics. For example, another of my interviewees commented: *"If you want to know what buildings are accessible, you need to go by the student route. The student route is focusing on whether the students can get into the lecture theatre not whether the lecturer can get onto the stage"* (Academic 11). Hence, Stone et al. (2013) characterize chronically ill academics as "unexpected workers in an able-bodied work environment" (p. 151).

Research demonstrates that it is more difficult for disabled employees to attain senior or leadership positions, with a "glass ceiling" hindering promotion and advancement. In addition, Roulestone and Williams (2014) describe the impact of "glass partitions". They explain that disabled managers are often reluctant to change roles (on an internal or external basis) as role change or organizational restructure increases the potential for disability to be discussed with subsequent stigma or discrimination. As described by one disabled manager, "The thought of having a new manager or management reporting system is pretty horrific for me ... I would hate to have to begin to explain how my mental health and my role can sit together" (Roulestone & Williams, 2014, pp. 22–23). These 'glass partition' issues are likely to impact disabled faculty experiencing university restructures. Further, academics are often expected to be geographically mobile. For example, they may obtain a series of short-term post-doc research positions before securing a permanent lectureship. There is, however, little consideration of the impact of role change on disabled academics, in relation to potential stigma or discrimination, issues such as disrupted access to medical care, or the long-term career outcomes for those unable to routinely change roles.

As discussed in Chapter 3, higher education is a competitive and challenging profession. Disabled employees are often assumed to be less competent or capable than their non-disabled colleagues (see *Perceived competence* section, this chapter). Disabled faculty also report that they are perceived to be less valuable and capable than their non-disabled counterparts, and as a consequence they are expected to be "grateful" for their position (Opini, 2010). Both overt (e.g. limited promotion or development opportunities) and subtle (e.g. contributions ignored in meetings or social exclusion) forms of discrimination occur. There may be particular issues in relation to academia and mental health. As Academic 3 explained, her colleague's openness about mental health was criticized: "*Someone said to him, 'you know, your mind is your living, why would you admit that there's something wrong with it?'.*"

Similarly, Academic 4 reflected on her experience of mental health: "*There's such a kudos attached to intelligence and brainpower and intellectualism. If you say, 'My brain is negatively impacted by this illness that I have', it's like this kind of inferiority thing associated with that. So I do think academia is a bit of a ... it is a bit of a kind of case apart, where there's like, an extra layer of stuff that comes along with saying, you have a problem with your mind.*" Furthermore, though personal experience of disability may enhance academic understanding, faculty whose disability informs their research or practice may be vulnerable to negative judgement. For example, as a mental health service user/survivor working in academia, Carr (2019) reports becoming the subject of the following Twitter comment after a conference: "It looks like Dr Sarah Carr ... has made quite a career out of 'lived experience' in MH. Clever cookie. Fleecing the system" (Carr, 2019, p. 1142).

Such attitudes can have a considerable impact on disabled academics. As described by one disabled faculty member, "I am not the world's most self-confident person and have a tendency to internalise the stigmatising narratives around disability, part of the reason for my initial denial. Over time, the daily passive aggression (long glances, patronising language) has led to a sense of less and a degree of isolation" (Mellifont et al., 2019, p. 1189). This academic further commented: "There have even been instances where people without disability see themselves as more deserving (of tasks/opportunities) – a blind belief that they can do better because they are not encumbered by disability. This is one of the symptoms of cookie-cutter recruitment and a lack of true diversity" (Mellifont et al., 2019, p. 1189).

Some academics may also feel compelled to challenge the stigma and stereotypes encountered. As described by one academic, "My experiences within the academy were, and continue to be, drenched with numerous deliberate efforts to counteract disability-related stereotypes" (Lourens, 2020, p. 1207). Similarly, an academic I interviewed stated: "*I think there's a huge misunderstanding and stigma around it. And you know, and to an extent, I try and sort of educate people a little bit*" (Academic 8). This is not an easy process, however, with those who challenge stereotypes and discrimination vulnerable to further mistreatment and isolation.

Securing workplace accommodations is also difficult. The stress associated with seeking accommodations and the time and energy required from the employee may be a deterrent, particularly if stress exacerbates symptoms. One faculty member commented, "I'm just too tired right now to look into it" (Stone et al., 2013, p. 160). Requests for workplace accommodations are often unsupported. One person recalled, "[O]ne of the ... faculty actually said to me, 'Well, maybe you need to think of a different career'. I thought, 'oh boy, aren't you going to tell me first we should try some accommodations?'" (Stone et al., 2013, p. 163). Managers may be especially unwilling to reduce workloads. As described by one academic: *"if I said to my institute that I needed to reduce some of the commitments that I have, because I'm just too tired to fill them, they would be probably going down the route of I'm unable to fulfil my contractual duties. And I know that because I've been involved in managing another person who's got anxiety and depression and can't do some of the things. She's got some physical disabilities and that's what they're doing, is trying to get her dismissed"* (Academic 5).

Summary

People with disabilities that are visible or known to others are at risk of stigma and discrimination. Such mistreatment extends to the workplace, with disabled people experiencing discrimination at each stage of the recruitment, promotion, and retention process. Disabled academics report a range of negative experiences, including difficulties accessing the required workplace accommodations. The stigma and discrimination associated with disability must be addressed on a societal level in order to support disabled employees.

Measuring attitudes towards disability

A number of standardized measures have been created to measure attitudes (both positive and negative) about disability. For example, Popovich et al. (2003) developed the 88-item Disability Questionnaire to assess (1) beliefs about what constitutes a disability, (2) affective reactions to working with people with disabilities, and (3) beliefs about the reasonableness of workplace accommodations. For the first subscale, respondents identify the conditions (from a list of 42) that they believe to be disabilities. The researchers identified considerable variation in what is perceived to constitute a disability, with physical and sensory-motor conditions (e.g. impaired hearing) more likely to be classified as a disability than psychological conditions (e.g. schizophrenia). For the affective reaction subscale (21 items) and reasonableness of workplace accommodations subscale (25 items), participants indicate their agreement with a series of statements (e.g. "I am uncomfortable with the idea of sharing my work space with a disabled person") or the extent to which the listed accommodation is reasonable.

Copeland et al. (2010) further examined the structure of the 21-item affective reaction subscale. Three dimensions were identified: (1) negative cognitive and affective reactions (e.g. "Working with an individual with a disability would increase my workload"), (2) positive attitudes towards accommodating co-workers with disabilities (e.g. "I would be willing to cover work for a co-worker with a disability who had to miss work because of their disability"), and (3) positive attitudes towards equal treatment of people with disabilities in the workplace (e.g. "It is important to have workers with disabilities in the workforce"). Such measures provide important opportunities to assess attitudes and monitor the effectiveness of interventions intended to support equality, diversity, and inclusion initiatives. Of course, participants may not respond truthfully to self-report questionnaires and observational methods are also important. For example, Cahill and Eggleston (1995) used participant observation to examine public assistance of wheelchair users.

Sexual orientation and stigma

Stigma is not restricted to mental and physical health conditions. Academics may experience stigma and discrimination centred on other protected characteristics such as ethnicity, religion, or sexual orientation. For example, heterosexism stigmatizes non-heterosexual behaviour and identity, and enforces strict adherence to gender role stereotypes. Heterosexist acts such as refusing to acknowledge homosexual relationships, derogatory jokes, and overt physical or verbal aggression may each impact on LGBTQ+ academics. Silverschanz et al. (2008) report that heterosexist harassment is widespread in academia, with negative impacts on both homosexual and heterosexual students. However, comparatively little research has addressed this in relation to academics rather than student populations.

Research that has addressed this subject indicates that the relative invisibility of homosexuality, interpersonal discomfort, and pressure to "cover" one's sexual orientation are more common than overt hostility (Bilimoria & Stewart, 2009), and the need to navigate potentially difficult interactions and anticipation of rejection by colleagues and peers may cause considerable stress (Dozier, 2015). As a consequence, gay and lesbian faculty report restricting interactions with colleagues to professional rather than personal subjects, contributing to social isolation and anxiety (Bilimoria & Stewart, 2009). As commented by one academic, "I personally believe that academe is one of the most difficult places to be out because though we are often enveloped by a (supposedly) liberal environment, heterosexism has an insidious way of permeating that seemingly accepting exterior and striking at the core of people's deepest fears" (McNaron, 1997, p. 6).

Addressing the career consequences for lesbian, gay, and bisexual academics in one subject discipline, Taylor and Raeburn (1995) focus on the activities of the Lesbian and Gay Caucus that has challenged sexual orientation-based stigma and advocated for equal treatment. They report that those participating in this form of political activism are more vulnerable to discrimination in recruitment and promotion. They are also more likely to be excluded from professional or social networks, to have their work devalued, and to experience harassment or intimidation. To reduce stigma and discrimination, it is important to consider the wider university culture. For example, an inclusive campus environment and opportunities for LGBTQ+ networking are important facilitators for the development of an academic career (Sanchez et al., 2015).

One barrier to inclusivity and acceptance is the adoption by some universities, particularly in North America, of "honour codes". These codes of conduct may include references to both academic (e.g. plagiarism) and non-academic (e.g. alcohol consumption) behaviour and universities with a religious focus are especially likely to refer to sexual behaviour. For example, in 2021 the Code of Conduct at Messiah University (Pennsylvania) includes: "Sexually inappropriate behavior. This includes overly intimate sexual behavior, sexual intercourse outside of marriage, same sex sexual expression and the use or distribution of pornography. Students who experience same sex attraction or identify as gay or lesbian are expected to refrain from same sex sexual expression."

Similarly, in 2021 the Code of Conduct for Regent University (Virginia) states: "Sexual Conduct. Regent University fully accepts the teachings of the traditional Biblical view with regard to the goodness of heterosexual marriage as God's intended context for complete sexual expression to occur (Gen. 2:21–24)," and "Sexual misconduct that is prohibited includes disorderly conduct or lewd, indecent, or obscene conduct or expression, involvement with pornography, premarital sex, adultery, homosexual conduct or any other conduct that violates Biblical standards." The honour codes are traditionally targeted at student behaviour, although institutions that are hostile to homosexual students are also likely to also be hostile to LGBTQ+ academics.

3 Academic culture and context

Disability is an important subject to understand and address, regardless of the culture or context in which it is situated. It is, however, also important to consider the specific issues experienced by disabled people who are based within academia. This specialist contextual information allows us to identify the most problematic aspects of the prevailing academic culture and enables us to provide tailored advice and guidance to higher education institutions. Of particular relevance to academic culture are the use of performance metrics, long working hours, and temporary contracts that increasingly characterize the academic experience. These aspects of higher education increase the (perceived and actual) vulnerability of all faculty, but are especially problematic for those who are disabled. Therefore, this chapter addresses the Neoliberal academic culture that dominates modern higher education practice and the consequences of this culture for disabled academics.

Academic culture

Culture can be defined as "a system of inherited concepts expressed in symbolic forms by means of which people communicate, perpetuate, and develop their own knowledge about and attitudes toward life" (Geertz, 1973, p. 89). It shapes all aspects of our lives, from the routine to the remarkable, whether work-related or not. On a personal level, culture influences the food that we eat, the clothes that we wear, the way in which we form romantic relationships, and how we raise our children. In the workplace, culture creates traditions and customs that shape a wide range of attitudes and behaviour. Indeed, it does so at a national, sector, and institutional level. For example, whilst some companies have positioned themselves as relatively collaborative and informal, others are hierarchical and competitive. Unsurprisingly, these cultural practices have a considerable impact on our job satisfaction, organizational commitment, and employee health and wellbeing (e.g. Lok & Crawford, 2004).

The academic workplace is no exception to this type of cultural influence. Indeed, the academic culture shapes notions of both faculty and student success and the activities that are to be rewarded or encouraged. For example, one of the most prominent themes within the academic literature (and, perhaps, academia itself) has been the teaching vs. research debate. Although both activities are central to the academic role, the greater prestige of research compared with teaching is widely acknowledged. Hence, research outputs have a greater impact on faculty progression than teaching activities (Dobele & Rundle-Theile, 2015), and those wishing to progress within academia may feel compelled to focus on this area of their practice. Furthermore, only "legitimate" forms of research are accepted. As summarized by one academic: *"You might be a crap teacher, you might actually be only talking to 20 people who read the same journal that you do, whereas I might be doing a conference to thousands or a webinar to thousands, that changes lives. But because it's not in a paper with a reference at the end of it, that's not respected"* (Academic 2).

The emergence of Neoliberal ideology

> ... having a love of learning, a passion for teaching, and a commitment to intellectual integrity become relevant only insofar as they can be harnessed for the production process and repackaged as 'quality assured' ... outputs.
> (Roberts, 2007, p. 359)

In recent years, the most noticeable cultural shift that has impacted on higher education has been the emergence of Neoliberal ideology. Neoliberalism refers to "a theory of political economic practices that proposes that human well-being can best be advanced by liberating individual entrepreneurial freedoms and skills within an institutional framework characterized by strong private property rights, free markets, and free trade" (Harvey, 2005, p. 2). This Neoliberal culture places considerable importance on the economic climate, productivity, and quantification. In the context of higher education, Neoliberal culture is specifically characterized by the focus on individual, departmental, and institutional performance and the prominence of standardized metrics to quantify these outputs (Ball, 2012). Such measures are frequently employed to assess both academic (e.g. teaching and research activity) and student (e.g. performance and satisfaction) focused outcomes.

In Britain, the shift towards a Neoliberal educational ideology was exacerbated by the reduction in public funding (reflecting national austerity measures), rise in student tuition fees, and increased student numbers (often referred to as the "massification" of higher education). These issues have increased the extent to which potential students, funding agencies, and other interested parties make direct comparisons between institutions and have intensified competition within the sector. This competition has impacted on numerous higher education domains, including the recruitment of students, research funding applications, and appointment of high-profile "superstar" academics. Hence, higher education has arguably transformed from a collegial collaborative model to a managerial model which emphasizes performance appraisal and encourages competition between individual academics (Holmes & McElwee, 1995).

Performance metrics

> We are required to spend increasing amounts of our time in making ourselves accountable, reporting on what we do rather than doing it. There are new sets of skills to be acquired here – skills of presentation and of inflation, making the most of ourselves, making a spectacle of ourselves. (Ball, 2012, p. 19)

An environment in which academics must demonstrate their achievements in order to justify their position contributes to an emerging culture of surveillance, mistrust, and competition within academia. As one of my interviewees stated: "*It kind of brings out this really aggressively competitive streak, which is innate in all of us I think, but it's kind of the corporate environment that academia has now become*" (Academic 4). In Britain, frequently employed student experience or teaching-oriented performance metrics include the National Student Survey (NSS) and the Teaching Excellence Framework (TEF). Research-based metrics are also employed (such as the Research Excellence Framework, REF). Those who favour this type of performance assessment have typically argued that the use of standardized metrics and performance appraisal increases transparency and fairness, enhances course provision, and can increase faculty satisfaction and productivity (Reece et al., 2008). Indeed, an important feature of the Neoliberal university is "the re-invention of professionals themselves as units of resources whose performance and productivity must constantly be audited so that it can be enhanced" (Shore & Wright, 1999, p. 559).

However, whilst advocates of these measures often highlight the use of these metrics to reward performance, metrics can also be used in a punitive manner and may undermine educator confidence in their practice (Mercer-Mapstone et al., 2017; Moore & Kuol, 2005). In this manner, the performance-focused academic culture can limit innovative academic practice and constrain rather than promote creativity. In addition, academics who are subject to this type of assessment may simply shape their practice to the type of performance metric employed (Moya et al., 2015). For example, they may focus on the content that is popular (and hence improves student satisfaction) rather than material that has a sound pedagogic basis that challenges student learning. Hence, the use of these metrics can encourage poor educational practice and lead to a distortion of the research or teaching agenda (Bridges, 2011; Holland et al., 2016). Indeed, the suggestion that increased assessment and quantification improves academia is often questioned. As stated by one professor, "There's a Danish proverb that says you don't fatten a pig by weighing it. And we are weighed far too often" (Sang et al., 2015, p. 244).

Giroux: Challenging the Neoliberal agenda

> Academic knowledge has been stripped of its value as a social good. To be relevant, and therefore adequately funded, knowledge has to justify itself in market terms or simply perish. (Giroux, 2014, p. 69)

Many educationalists have challenged the Neoliberal agenda. In particular, Giroux combines critical pedagogy and radical democracy to address the emergence of the Neoliberal university and criticize the banking approach to education in which information is "deposited" from teacher to student. Giroux (2014, 2015) argues that in recent years, educators have been relegated to the role of technicians, forced to simply transfer information to students and "teach to the test". In addition, educators are pressured to focus on employability-related issues that prepare students for their future role in the economy rather than the development of critical thinking skills that prepare students for engagement in a democracy. Specifically, he states: "Teachers are stripped of their worth and dignity by being forced to adopt an educational vision and philosophy that has little respect for the empowering possibilities of either knowledge or critical classroom practices" (Giroux, 2015, p. 3).

Giroux is especially critical of standardized metrics that are continually used to quantify and critique the performance of students and educators. He refers to this as "a mindless infatuation with metrics and modes of testing" (Giroux, 2015, p. 3) and proposes that educators move away from a banking model of education in order to focus on the aspects of teaching and learning that promote social action and agency. To some extent, Giroux is sympathetic to educators who are increasingly subject to surveillance and audit. He also recognizes the pressures faced by academics such as excessive workloads and the increased use of fixed-term contracts. Despite these pressures, Giroux remains critical of educators who do not challenge the Neoliberal system. He states: "too many academics have become overly comfortable with the corpo-ratization of the university and the new regimes of Neoliberal governance. Chasing after grants, promotions, and conventional research outlets, many academics have retreated from larger public debates and refused to address urgent social problems" (Giroux, 2014, p. 17).

The academic role

> "I feel like I'm hanging by a frayed thread right now. There is this kind of posturing about overwork, and workaholism, which is toxic, and it's addictive. But because it's socially acceptable to be a workaholic, because it works in the interest of the institution and the government, it's like you get your little pat on the head, and it's fine. And it's like, no, there's actually something seriously dysfunctional about that." (Academic 4)

The academic role encompasses a range of complex activities and responsibilities centred on teaching, research, and administration. Academic roles are also characterized by excessive workloads. Indeed, these have become normalized in academia. In one study, approximately 90% of academics reported working after hours and over two-thirds of those questioned worked more than ten hours beyond their full-time hours (Houston et al., 2006). Intense workloads are related to stress (Mkumbo, 2014) and people with excessive working hours and a poor work–life balance are less likely to remain in academia (Lindfelt et al., 2018). Hence, workloads impact on both individual professionals and the wider education sector. Though technology may provide faculty with greater flexibility, increased opportunities to work from home have further blurred boundaries between work and home. As a consequence, it may be difficult for academics to "switch off" with, for example, the tendency to send or respond to emails on mobile phones increasing expectations that people are always available (Currie & Eveline, 2011). In addition to the implicit or explicit expectations that relate to academic workloads, faculty may also work long hours through a sense of commitment to their work and academic fulfilment. As stated by one early career academic, "I'm not really too bothered if I spend a lot of time at work because I enjoy it: it's who I am, it's a big part of my identity" (Cannizzo et al., 2019, p. 258).

Of course, issues arise when faculty are pressured into long working hours in order to "keep up" and remain competitive in the demanding academic environment. As summarized by one of my interviewees: *"So there's, on the one hand, an acknowledgement that people should only be working, you know, a certain number of hours every week and should have a work–life balance and should be able to work when they're well and got the energy. But on the other hand, you are actually judged against people who have more energy and can work till one o'clock in the morning"* (Academic 5). Though academic workloads and whether academics should engage in these extended working hours are important issues in themselves, it is important to highlight the impact of this culture on faculty who are unable to perform in this manner. For example, it may be especially difficult for faculty with children or caring responsibilities to adopt these schedules (Hardy et al., 2018). Increased workloads also impact on many academics with disabilities, particularly those with energy-limiting conditions.

As described by one academic: *"There was a good point when it was all being managed. And it was all working out well. It was about probably about four or five years ago now though. I got back in the swing of things and I was actually thinking, 'Okay, well, I'm going to do this research', I mean ... I was getting some really good invites to present at conferences and being able to find the time to do those. Because I had to have extra time, either side of the conference, because of the impact the travel had. And I managed to sort all of that out. And then, I don't think I've changed, but the demands of academia have changed, which has then meant that all of those, I'd say more that the positive sides of the role, have actually just been squeezed to the point where they're virtually non-existent. Now, I'm just carrying on trying to consciously juggle, keep plates flying around, and hoping that none of them drop. Or when they do drop, I can sort them out pretty quickly"* (Academic 1).

Excessive workloads can impact on the health and wellbeing of disabled faculty, particularly when there are no accommodations or adjustments for their health status. As described by one of my interviewees: *"When I came back from my sick leave, there was just, there was no change in my workload. It was like, 'Oh there, there [moves as if you would comfort a child] but we're expecting you to do a normal full workload, because the business model is like, it's necessary, business wise.' And then if I'd refuse, then I could be taken to a tribunal for not doing my job properly, do you know what I mean. Then I could lose my job. So of course, I'm sort of stuck in this situation where it's really bad for my health, because they won't make any concessions at all, even though it's a disability"* (Academic 4).

In many institutions, workload allocation models have been introduced to regulate academic workloads, with pre-determined hours assigned to specific roles and responsibilities. It is typically argued that these promote fairness and transparency. However, these workload models often fail to capture the range of tasks undertaken by academics or the time required to complete them (Miller, 2019). For example, one early career academic explained that workload policies were reasonable but, "If you're going to do the job properly and at a high level and if you're teaching, get the student evaluations that say you're a good teacher and play a big role in your advancement, then you have to do a whole lot of extra work" (Cannizzo et al., 2019, p. 258). These workload models are also vulnerable to abuse. As explained by another of my interviewees: *"What's happened in effect is we were all on about 120, 130% of the workload allocation model a couple of years ago. So rather than actually doing anything about it, they just altered the criteria for the workload model and the amount of time that you've got for that. So that now, most of us are on between 80 and 90%, but actually doing considerably more than the last couple of years"* (Academic 1).

In recent years, the proportion of temporary or precarious contracts within academia has also risen. Academics on temporary contracts are less satisfied with their academic position (Castellacci & Vinas-Bardolet, 2020). However, the impact of job security extends beyond the academic role. Those employed on temporary contracts are less able to purchase their own home and this insecurity negatively impacts on the stability of family life (Waaijer et al., 2017). It is, therefore, not surprising that temporary contracts are associated with increased employee stress and anxiety. Indeed, Loveday (2018) conceptualizes anxiety as both a symptom of precarious working conditions and a "tactic" adopted by Neoliberal academia to control, regulate, and discipline the behaviour of employees.

The use of short-term temporary contracts, often requiring candidates to be geographically mobile, is especially problematic for some academics (e.g. those with caring responsibilities). For disabled faculty, the use of temporary contracts requiring movement to a new institution and/or area can disrupt the consistency of health care and workplace accommodations. For example, faculty may be unable to receive accommodations in their new role before assessment at the new institution. Reliance on short-term contracts is also likely to cause considerable anxiety for those working in countries where access to medical insurance and treatment is dependent on full-time employment.

Ableism and disability in academia

The pressures faced by academics are clear. Faculty are expected to produce both more outputs and higher quality outputs (Soliman & Soliman, 1997) and this academic culture is inherently unhealthy. As stated by Parizeau et al. (2016),

"We experience academic cultures and practices that valorize overwork, including expressions of martyrdom, talking about not sleeping or eating and about working all of the time, an expectation of always being available for work purposes." They continue:

> "Some of us have experienced toxic workplaces that do not always manifest themselves in visible, quantifiable, or written forms, but through regular, routine, or everyday micropolitics and microaggressions that are often difficult for those experiencing them to name and where competition, insularity, and insecurity can escalate to bullying, sabotage, backstabbing, and character assassination" (pp. 197–198).

The academic culture places significant pressure on academics to conform to this standard. Academics often report that the culture of long working hours and intense productivity leads to feelings of guilt or inadequacy and a fear of falling behind their colleagues. As described by one academic, "the level of guilt that one experiences sometimes is relentless … there is always something you should be doing in academia, I think it is relentless. I've had to work very hard, and I'm still not there, at letting go of some of that guilt" (Hawkins et al., 2014, p. 336).

The Neoliberal academic culture is especially difficult for those with disabilities. For example, England (2016) describes the extent to which bipolar status has impacted on time management and productivity moving "between lacklustre and stellar performance" (p. 228). In a competitive and performance-driven environment that closely monitors the activities and achievement of employees, disabled academics may feel pressure to "prove themselves" in an attempt to overcompensate for their disabled status and guard against the discrimination experienced by people with disabilities (Schwartz & Elder, 2018; Shier et al., 2009). Indeed, the emphasis on productivity and performance is inherently ableist, suggesting that individuals can and should be able to work excessive hours and excel in both teaching and research without any impact on their personal health and wellbeing (Tuinamuana, 2016). This is compounded by stereotyped perceptions of disabled people as less capable or productive than their non-disabled peers (Hughes, 2009).

Ableism, defined as "a pervasive system of discrimination and exclusion that oppresses people who have mental, emotional and physical disabilities" (Rauscher & McClintock, 1996, p. 198) creates an environment that is often hostile to them. There has been a paucity of research addressing ableism within academia (Mellifont et al., 2019) and where such issues are discussed, they are often focused on disabled students or participants rather than academics with disabilities (e.g. Budge et al., 2016; Saltes, 2020a). For recent exceptions focused on the ableism experienced by disabled academics, see Brown and Leigh (2020) and Brown (2021).

Although disability impacts on the faculty experience and disabled academics are underrepresented within the sector (Brown & Leigh, 2018), ableism appears to be more tolerated in higher education than discrimination against other protected characteristics. As described by one of my interviewees: *"Nobody but nobody would tolerate us having a whites only campus, there* would be horror, it would be all over the news, there would be pickets, and rightly so on that disgraceful set of affairs if we didn't allow black people into buildings. But we've got a campus where our shared teaching spaces is 0.5%, so 99.5% of our shared teaching spaces on campus, disabled people can't get into" (Academic 10).

Impairment interacts with all aspects of the academic role, including the aforementioned long working hours. As described by another of my interviewees: "*I would have to sometimes travel for up to five hours a day ... it was really, really difficult. I didn't really manage it very well, and I take full responsibility for that. Like, I'm someone who is a doer. And I'm not very good at taking time for myself. So I just kind of run myself ragged for kind of three, four days and just try and cope the best I can*" (Academic 8). In part this may reflect the pressures placed on faculty members and the precarity of academia. For example, this academic also stated: "*It's really difficult. If you're on a project, it can really easily just run away with you, you know. I was the only researcher and I really wanted the project to succeed, not just, you know, altruistic reasons, but because of myself, you know. I needed a job and ultimately if the project didn't work and the funding goes, then your job goes*" (Academic 8).

Disability may also change the way that faculty engage with their work. As described by one academic I interviewed: "*A lot of the performative stuff that people tend to do like having blogs, Twitter accounts, um disseminating ideas in the media, making sure that they get their stuff out there in terms of impact. I can't do that kind of stuff. I tend to tend to ... it means that I work on my own quite a bit to be honest, because collaborations involve an awful lot of the pre-research steps. They complicate the planning because somebody's got to allocate roles, you've got to agree who's doing it, you've got to do the network for the partnerships. Whereas if I just sit down and do my research by myself, then I can produce my research without having to go through all of those other performative steps which ... I mean that has an impact, it's quite marginalizing, you know*" (Academic 10).

Of course, some elements of the academic role may be more problematic than others. For example, academic conferences can be especially difficult. To attend conferences, faculty may be required to travel long distances and navigate a range of transport that may not be accessible. Such events are also exhausting for those with energy-limiting conditions. Whilst attending the conference, there are often few opportunities for those who may be noise or light sensitive to rest or to seek the respite required when feeling anxious. In this manner, tasks which may be a routine – or even pleasurable – part of the academic role for those without a disability (and provide important opportunities to network with colleagues) can be challenging for those with a disability, requiring additional time and resources. Furthermore, the dissemination of research findings through conference attendance is often included in academic progression or promotion criteria. As discussed by one of my interviewees: "*I couldn't go without a carer. And nobody is going to pay for that. So that kind of thing with minimal budgets means that I have to somehow disseminate research, prove that I'm doing research, because there are no reasonable adjustments made around that kind of thing, despite the fact that I can't get to conferences. So I'm forever looking out for webinars to see if you can do bits of networking like that, you know"* (Academic 10).

For many subjects, fieldwork is central to the discipline. Fieldwork can be problematic for academics and students with disabilities (Hall & Healey, 2005). For example, travel may disrupt treatment regimens and there may be little privacy for rest or recovery. In addition, the field sites may be less accessible for those with mobility issues, and increased time with others in an unfamiliar environment may be overwhelming for individuals with sensory or mental health conditions. These issues are, of course, further compounded by difficulty engaging with normal coping mechanisms (e.g. distance from social support networks). Tucker and Horton (2019) document the difficulties encountered by academics with mental health conditions when engaging with residential fieldwork. Academics reported: "Staff and students continue to be expected to work between 8am–11pm on physical geography fieldcourses. This concerns me greatly … I have never, either as staff or student, come home well from a residential fieldcourse" (p. 89). Furthermore, "Fieldtrips are very isolating. I find that kind of intense scrutiny – being under the gaze of students and colleagues – difficult to cope with. I just want to get away from them!" (p. 90).

Adjustments and accommodations

Though institutions have a legal obligation to support disabled employees and make reasonable adjustments, many universities do not have a formal accommodation policy and do not make appropriate adjustments (Saltes, 2020b). For example, academics may be scheduled to teach in rooms that are not accessible or may not be given sufficient time to process important documentation. Indeed, academics with disabilities appear to be less supported than disabled students. As summarized by Smith and Andrews (2015), "Higher education institutions are often well prepared in terms of accommodation policies and practices for disabled students. Ironically, campuses are often not prepared once disabled academics return as faculty" (p. 1521). As described by one of my interviewees: "*I get sent Learning Support plans all the time for people who have mental health conditions. Students who have mental health conditions, there is a lot of extra time they're allowed, you know, to be absent if health is bad. But I'm not given any of that, even the acknowledgement, like it's just not there. It's a total double standard*" (Academic 4).

Adjustments to academic workloads appear to be especially problematic. One academic I interviewed explained: "*I went to see my line manager and said, 'Look, I don't want to be signed off again. But is there anything we can do? Because I'm really, really concerned for my mental health, like, I'm not doing very well.' And he just said, 'Well, we can't have you doing 80% of what we're paying you for now, can we?'*" (Academic 4). Difficulties also frequently arose because adjustments were dependent on the approval of a line manager. For example, one academic stated: "*I think if you're lucky to have a line manager who's understanding, then you're lucky. And if you're not, you can forget it, you don't get anything*"; "*Occupational health have been excellent, but it's down to the management team in our school to decide whether or not the reasonable adjustments that occupational health have recommended are acceptable*" (Academic 1).

In practice, where accommodations *are* provided, it is often disabled faculty that are required to arrange this support, with little institutional guidance (Waterfield et al., 2018). For example, academics may be responsible for arranging their interpreters and checking that assigned teaching spaces are accessible. This has a substantial impact on the workload of disabled academics (Hannam-Swain, 2018). As described by one of my interviewees: "*This is something that people don't realize, that sheer burden of disability admin. Over the course of this doctorate, I have lost over a month of full-time working hours, just to disability admin. People have no idea*" (Academic 12). As a consequence, academics with disabilities have less time available to complete other academic tasks (putting them at a disadvantage when competing with non-disabled colleagues) or for their personal lives (which impacts on their mental and physical wellbeing). Indeed, Inckle (2018) describes "the extra work which I have to undertake which is neither paid, nor acknowledged in my workload and which places significant physical, emotional and mental burdens on me" (p. 1372). She further explains that this is particularly intense when adopting a new position that requires adjustment to the new role, completion of mandatory training, and preparation of new teaching materials. This is, of course, particularly important in the context of increasing temporary contracts and excessive workloads described previously in the chapter (e.g. Houston et al., 2006).

It is, not just the amount of time required to make such arrangements that places an additional burden on disabled academics. For example, Inckle (2018) describes the extent to which negotiating with Human Resources, Facilities Management, etc. "require a huge amount of emotional labour and resilience on my part, which is compounded by hostile, patronising and sometimes bullying responses from university staff when I progress them" (p. 1375). To some extent, the concept of "adjustments" may itself be problematic. It is reminiscent of the medical model that represents people with disabilities as "problems to be solved". Instead, institutions should create an inclusive and accessible environment rather than adjusting the inaccessible university to accommodate individual employees. Adjustments made on a case-by-case basis can make disabled employees uncomfortable and require disclosure by the disabled employee that is often problematic. For example, it may be difficult for those without a formal medical diagnosis to receive support. This reactive ableist approach characterizes many university processes.

As described by one of my interviewees: "*And I'd had this discussion with HR. And their response was, 'No, we don't do it that way. But if you wanted to put in for a promotion, you'd fill everything out and then there's a section on mitigating circumstances that you could then fill in to explain why you haven't met the criteria for promotion.' And I'm like, that's totally wrong. Actually, that's an ablest view. So you've got to basically set yourself up to fail. And for it to be turned down, and then explain why it shouldn't be turned down*"

(Academic 1). In addition, non-disabled employees may resent changes to existing policy and practice: *"They would make comments in committee meetings like, 'Oh well, we can't do this anymore like this, because of [gives name].' And they were so horrible to her that she has left the university and taken another role"* (Academic 5).

Academia and the COVID-19 pandemic

The impact of the COVID-19 pandemic on the education sector cannot be overstated. Academics and professional services staff transitioned to online teaching, assessment, and student support immediately. This transmission typically required the development or adaptation of teaching and assessment materials suitable for online learning, engagement with new technology, and a substantial range of administrative tasks (e.g. consultation with professional bodies) to introduce the required modular and programme changes. At the same time, faculty revised their research agendas to address pandemic-specific issues and accommodate restrictions on face-to-face data collection. Indeed, academics frequently experienced professional and societal pressure to produce and disseminate pandemic-specific research (Carusi et al., 2020). This all occurred during a period of intense stress and anxiety, with some subject disciplines, such as Nursing, supporting faculty and students who also operated on the frontline of COVID care (Hayter & Jackson, 2020).

Emerging evidence suggests that the COVID-19 pandemic has exacerbated existing inequalities within the education sector, with respect to student, researcher, and educator progression. For example, numerous higher education institutions moved to implement redundancies and cease the recruitment of new staff or the renewal of existing temporary contracts, citing a reduced income (e.g. loss of international student fees). This has disproportionately impacted on early career academics, who may be unable to secure an academic contract (Kinikoglu & Can, 2021). As summarized by Park (2020), "Faced with university closures, hiring freezes, and a general lack of support and benefits, an entire generation of postdocs and their knowledge and skills may be lost to academia without intervention" (p. 543).

Female academics with children have also been disproportionately impacted by the COVID-19 pandemic (Cardel et al., 2020; Crook, 2020), with caregiving and home-schooling responsibilities limiting the hours available for academic work and subsequent productivity. This is evident in fewer journal publications by and grant submissions for female academics (Krukowski et al., 2020). If this gender disparity is not acknowledged and addressed in recruitment and promotion decisions, COVID-19 will continue to impede the career progression of female academics. Indeed, a range of recommendations have been made (e.g. extending grant periods) to support female academics negatively disadvantaged by the COVID-19 pandemic (Cardel et al., 2020), though the extent to which these will be implemented remains unclear.

People with disabilities have been perhaps most severely impacted by the pandemic. COVID-19 presents specific risks and challenges to the disabled community (Jalali et al., 2020; Kuper et al., 2020). In particular, whilst disabled people are at greater risk of morbidity and mortality from COVID-19, they may be de-prioritized for medical intervention and encouraged to sign "do not resuscitate" orders (Armitage & Nellums, 2020). In addition, the closure of non-essential services and diversion of medical resources including personnel to COVID-19 has reduced access to routine medical treatment, support, and rehabilitation (Lazzerini et al., 2020). Furthermore, though many people with disabilities have been required to "shield" for extended periods due to their increased risk of infection, social or physical distancing can be difficult for those who rely on the support of carers. As a consequence, people may be required to consider both the risk of infection and need for care when making decisions about their health and wellbeing.

These issues also affect disabled academics, particularly if they do not have access to supportive equipment or accommodations when working at home. Indeed, the move to home working may have had a considerable impact on employee occupational health (Bouziri et al., 2020). Although the pandemic presents challenges, it also offers the opportunity to consider alternative ways of working that are more accessible to the disabled community. Hannam-Swain and Bailey (2021) provide an autoethnographic account of COVID-19 as a disabled lecturer working in higher education in the UK. They highlight the lessons that may be taken from the pandemic (and associated changes in working practice) for accessibility and supporting disabled academics, students, and professional services staff. Hannam-Swain and Bailey (2021) state, "as we emerge from this period of crisis, we need to use these experiences as leverage for positive change; for designing ways of teaching and learning that accommodate everyone, rather than getting swept up in an unthinking pursuit of returning to 'business as usual'" (p. 1).

One significant difference for disabled academics working from home during the pandemic has been the provision of greater support for this mode of working. As outlined by one academic I interviewed: *"Oh my God, working from home has been amazing. I tried it once before and it didn't work fundamentally because the office wasn't set up to allow it. I do coding and to do this coding I need access to the data ... And getting remote access to it was extraordinarily difficult and extraordinarily slow to the point where you know, at times I've typed D, I'd have to wait a few seconds for it to come up on screen and it was just so frustrating to try and interact with it remotely. And they literally just, and there's a bit of me that feels guilty for how angry I feel at this, that they just sort of flipped a switch and made it work for everyone"* (Academic 11).

Reflection on the impact of the pandemic is not, of course, limited to the provision for disabled faculty. Corbera et al. (2020) encourage academics to foster a culture of care, focus on what is most important, and ensure that academic practice is "more respectful and sustainable" (p. 191). They suggest that the pandemic provides an opportunity to reflect on education and resist the Neoliberalization of academia, instead focusing on personal and collective wellbeing. They recognize the variation in lockdown experiences and suggest that we must acknowledge and act upon inequalities. For example, whilst some people have a safe and supportive home-working environment, others may not and limited economic resources may limit access to a high-speed internet connection or IT equipment, impacting on their ability to complete academic activities. Corbera et al. (2020) state, "When the COVID-19 crisis fades away, which it will, we have a chance to make academia a more ethical, empathetic, and thus rewarding profession" (p. 196).

There is, of course, no easy solution and the measures introduced to lessen the impact of the COVID-19 pandemic may be detrimental for some academic groups. For example, some journals have temporarily paused the processing of new article submissions as a public rejection of "academic normalcy". Whilst this reinforces the message that academics should not be expected to produce and publish as they would in a non-COVID-19 environment, this may negatively impact on those such as final-year PhD students or fixed contract academics who have limited time to secure a new position and are attempting to enhance their portfolio (Corbera et al., 2020). It is, therefore, essential that the impact of potential changes to policy or practice are considered with respect to equality, diversity, and inclusion. Indeed, this will be even more important as the full impact of long COVID emerges.

Summary

To conclude, academia represents a demanding and competitive environment in which the performance of faculty is closely monitored. In this context, disabled academics experience a number of disadvantages. In particular, they may not receive the accommodations required to fulfil their role and are often compared with non-disabled colleagues who are not required to spend time arranging accommodations and may be more able to engage in activities such as conference attendance and long working hours. Addressing negative aspects of academic culture is important for the wellbeing of all educators, but especially important for the health and inclusion of disabled academics.

4 Invisible disabilities and the decision to disclose

Disability-oriented research (including research addressing the experiences of disabled students and faculty) has typically focused on visible disabilities, such as those requiring the use of noticeable walking aids. In contrast, there has been far less attention to invisible conditions that may be concealed, such as depression or fibromyalgia. This chapter will consider the experience of people with invisible or non-visible disabilities and the decision to disclose or conceal such conditions. This includes disclosure to senior management, colleagues, and students. Both the positive (e.g. access to support) and negative (e.g. discrimination) consequences of disclosure will be considered, together with the lived experience of repeated disclosure.

Invisible disabilities and identity

Invisible or non-visible disabilities are impairments that are not immediately apparent, such as chronic fatigue syndrome, endometriosis, Crohn's disease, arthritis, and depression. Those with invisible stigma (e.g. invisible health conditions) are typically assumed to be "normal" (i.e. healthy). Therefore, faculty with non-visible conditions may be placed in a position of deciding whether to (a) challenge this assumption and self-disclose their stigmatized identity, or (b) attempt to "pass" as a person without a disability. Disclosure can be especially challenging if the disabled individual is not confident that their condition will be understood. The legitimacy or validity of many invisible conditions (e.g. chronic fatigue syndrome, Lyme disease) has been debated, encouraging suspicion and undermining the provision of support. Indeed, even medical professionals or members of a support group may query the validity of an invisible condition (Blanck, 2011).

Academics I interviewed contrasted the experience of visible or accepted impairments and invisible conditions. For example, one faculty member compared the responses she received following knee surgery with her everyday experience: "*I was actually feeling really good because I hadn't been at work and my energy levels were really high. So I was feeling really healthy. But the reaction from people was just totally different. It was very interesting, because* there was ... there was a lot more 'Oh, you okay? You doing alright?' And there was a lot more of a positive supportive reaction to that and I thought at the time, well if I came in and I'd really run out of energy, I'd sort of dragged myself in that hour and a half drive and had brain fog and was having difficulty articulating thoughts, would they have had that 'Oh, you feeling okay?' No, they wouldn't. I don't think they would, only a few of my very close colleagues would go, 'You're not having a good day today.' And everybody else would just think I'm not, erm well, I won't say negative thoughts, but it wouldn't be positive thoughts in terms of my contribution to what whatever I was doing at that time, or lack of it ... I don't think academia does get the invisible illness" (Academic 1).

As a consequence, those with invisible disabilities or difficult to diagnose conditions may be reluctant to disclose their impairment or doubt the validity of their own disability status (Fitzgerald & Paterson, 1995). One of my interviewees reported: "*I've withered on this for years. And I think whether or not I tick the box depends entirely on what sort of day I'm having. I think, particularly now, more recently, I think I would definitely think of myself as a person with a disability. For some reason disabled person sounds to me more severe. And also, like I don't have as much of a right to say that somehow*" (Academic 3). Another said: "*It depends who I'm with. I definitely don't mind saying I'm disabled, even though I do have imposter syndrome, about saying I'm disabled [laughs]. Because it's like this idea of I'm not disabled enough to, you know, I have the ... I go through these moments*" (Academic 9). Willingness to identify as disabled may also be influenced by the stigma surrounding (both visible and invisible) disability: "*It's a hard thing to admit, because our society says that disabled people are worth less. And you know, we don't have happy narratives for disabled people in our society, mostly because we treat them ... we treat us really badly*" (Academic 11).

The decision to identify as disabled often took a considerable length of time. For example, one faculty member explained: "*That's a journey and a process in itself. I'm at the end of a long process with that ... You don't want to see yourself like that. It is a new identity that you've got to take on, and one that you've got to adjust to*" (Academic 10). Increased symptom severity or formal diagnosis from a medical professional were especially important for identification and acceptance. For example, "*It's made a huge difference having a diagnosis. Because I did genuinely think of myself as somebody who was just lazy and ill-disciplined and a bit shit at a lot of things. And then I went, 'Oh, right. Oh, a condition right. Oh. It is actually genuinely more hard for me, right'*" (Academic 3).

It is important for those supporting disabled academics to recognize that people with disabilities may not necessarily identify as disabled or perceive themselves to be part of the disabled community (Prowse, 2009). Of course, identity has important consequences for access to accommodations and support. As one academic I spoke with explained: "*We had a situation at the beginning of COVID, where people could have equipment bought to their home.*

On the staff network, we had X amount of names. And then we said, 'is there any adaptive technology you have in your office that you need, but you need to let us know'. We probably had the same amount of people again saying, 'I'm not in the disabled network, but I need this.' It was back problems, it was wrist problems. And they didn't see themselves as disabled, because the term is not a pleasant term, in that sense. So people who do need additional support wouldn't say, 'I consider myself disabled', and therefore they don't get the network information, they don't get the support, because that's not a question that they want to say, 'Yes, I am, I consider myself disabled' to. I don't consider myself disabled, I consider myself as being very lucky that I'm creative, and I do things differently, but unless I tick that box, I'm not going to get anything, and that really annoys me" (Academic 2).

Self-disclosure

Self-disclosure has been defined as "the act of revealing personal information about oneself to another" (Collins & Miller, 1994, p. 457). Whilst self-disclosure is often discussed as an individual act, disclosure of a disability may involve a series of negotiations, discussions, and decisions rather than a single act of disclosure (Stanley et al., 2007). Similarly, people may choose to disclose their disabled status in one context but not another (Riddell & Weedon, 2014), demonstrating the complexity of the disclosure process. For example, an individual may disclose their condition to friends and family but not in the workplace. This disconnect can be problematic when people attempt to manage an identity that varies across contexts. For example, difficulties may arise if romantic partners are invited to a work function or if a friend begins work at the same organization. Disclosure may have important consequences for the individual. It is, therefore, important to consider the factors which may influence an individual's decision to self-disclose an invisible disability.

Academics may be especially reluctant to disclose. As summarized by one of my interviewees: *"There's such a culture of non-disclosure. There is such a culture of non-disclosure"* (Academic 12). This may impact on both those applying for academic roles and existing faculty. The same interviewee described her application for an academic role and her reluctance to disclose a condition that would have prioritized the application: *"There was a box and it said, 'Do you want to be prioritised for interview on disability grounds?' And I nearly didn't apply because of that box. Because I could not figure out what to say. And not in the sense of 'how do I word this', but simply, do I want you to know before you're interviewing me. Because you will, presumably because the search committee have to know that you must prioritise, that you have to interview this person ... And sort of thinking is there any point. Am I just gonna get interviewed for something they have absolutely no intention of employing me for?"* She further explained her decision to disclose only when a position had been secured: "*I do not disclose until I'm made an offer. Because at that point it's the deniability of it ... I don't want to disclose early because the prejudice 100% exists*" (Academic 12).

Factors influencing the decision to disclose

The disclosure process is complex, and both positive and negative outcomes may be anticipated. As one doctoral student explained, "The decision to disclose my disabilities to co-workers is always a fearful process filled with questions and uncertainties. For example, I often contemplate how knowledge about my disabilities will affect my career opportunities" (Solis, 2006, p. 152). Ragins (2008) argues that there are three primary antecedents to the disclosure of an invisible stigma (such as sexual orientation or health status): (1) internal psychological factors, (2) anticipated consequences of disclosure, and (3) environmental factors. These may, of course, only apply to those who recognize their own health condition as stigmatizing. A range of internal psychological factors may influence the self-disclosure process. According to self-verification theory, people are motivated to have others view them as they view themselves (Swann, 1983, 1987) and this affirms their identity and provides a sense of coherence. Therefore, where the disability is central to a person's self-concept, self-disclosure is more likely.

With regards to the positive consequences of disclosure, revealing a stigmatized identity may provide a sense of relief and reduce the stress associated with concealing this aspect of the self. It may also enhance self-esteem, facilitate emotional closeness in interpersonal relationships, and allow the person to identify and interact with others in a similar situation or with the same stigmatized identity. Access to practical support and legal protection from discrimination may also be dependent on self-disclosure. Indeed, for many people access to workplace accommodations is the primary motivation for disclosure. However, whilst disclosure may provide legal protection from discrimination or harassment, it may increase the likelihood of such behaviour. Those with disabilities are at increased risk of aggression from both strangers and non-strangers, including verbal abuse, violent crime, and sexual violence (see Ralph et al., 2016 for a review of disability hate crime). Exacerbating the impact of this violent behaviour, the severity of these crimes is often minimized, for example by referring to hate crime as bullying. Furthermore, victims may be re-traumatized by the judicial system, for example, by claims that disabled victims are "unreliable" witnesses.

In the workplace, employees are typically required to disclose in order to access workplace accommodations. However, employers often express concerns about the potential productivity, promotability, and flexibility of disabled employees (Hernandez et al., 2000). Hence, fear of discrimination (Munir et al., 2005) and the negative attitudes of others (Gilbride et al., 2000) represent significant barriers to disability disclosure. Indeed, the experience of requesting and securing workplace adjustments is highly varied and some employees report that negotiating accommodations led to bullying by line managers (Foster, 2007). In many respects, employees are reliant on the attitudes and awareness of individual line managers. In addition, colleagues are less likely to perceive accommodations as justified when disabilities are invisible or viewed as socially undesirable or self-caused (Colella, 2001) and may react negatively to accommodations if these are perceived as preferential treatment. Therefore, by requiring a person to disclose in order to receive accommodations, current practice draws attention to difference and may contribute to "othering".

Highlighting these concerns, one interviewee anticipated disclosing a worsening of symptoms to her line manager if she planned to become pregnant: *"If I decided to have a kid then I would have to come off most of my medication. Because it's linked to birth defects. So I would absolutely have to get rid of everything that is keeping me functional. How do you navigate that? You know 'um hi, hello HR. FYI I am in advance gonna have to stop taking the medication, that means that I sleep, that means I'm in significantly less pain over time. That means that, of course, I can't sleep, I can't stay awake during the day. So FYI, I am in advance gonna, for an indefinite period of time, because you can't plan things like conception, I'm gonna be wildly less productive, because of a choice that I've deliberately even actively made' ... I have no idea how I'm going to have that conversation with any employer"* (Academic 12).

Environmental factors may include the presence of others with similarly stigmatizing conditions, supportive relationships, and institutional support. For example, employees may feel more empowered to disclose if they have job security and some organizations and industries may be perceived as more open and accepting (Clair et al., 2005). As described by another of my interviewees, the disclosure process can be stressful: *"I wouldn't have felt comfortable because I would have been, I would have felt like I was sticking my head above the parapet and exposing ... because of all the constant threats. ... we're kind of constantly having an axe hanging over us. And we're in deficit, which the university likes to keep reminding us of and every time we lose somebody, they won't even pay for part-time teaching because of the deficit. And it's like, but we are skeleton staff as it is. We're all at breaking point. Even people who don't have mental illnesses are like really, really struggling. And it's like, this is just so hideously unsustainable and aggressive. I'm already working in that environment. If I'd said 'Oh, by the way, I have this disability. How about you reduce my workload?', they would have been ... I was just really worried about what would happen"* (Academic 4).

Wider social, cultural, and political issues may also inform the decision process. For example, Vickers (1997) suggests that the capitalist emphasis on individual productivity and efficiency encourages employees to conceal invisible health conditions. As a consequence, people may feel more confident disclosing a disability if they have "proven" their capability or commitment to the organization. For example, one of my interviewees stated: *"And I think, because I'd almost proved that I was a hard worker, and that I wasn't someone* who was taking the mick. Which, you shouldn't have to prove that. That's not a bar that should be set. But when I kind of said to him, I need to work from home today, he kind of understood that I'd reached a limit. And kind of, you know what that meant" (Academic 8).

The nature of the condition itself may also influence the decision process. For example, it may be more difficult for a person to self-disclose if there is no definitive test for their condition or if they do not have a formal diagnosis. Similarly, people may be reluctant to disclose if they fear that their condition will be misunderstood or that the validity of the condition will be questioned. For example, chronic fatigue syndrome has been frequently dismissed in the media as 'yuppie flu'. One interviewee stated: "*I worried about changing job and moving from [names city] to [names city]. And because it's like a whole new set of people that you've kind of, almost feels like you've got to convince them you know that this is a real thing*" (Academic 8). In contrast, people may be more likely to disclose if they potentially require support in a medical emergency or where self-disclosure is essential for management of the condition at work (Beatty, 2001). For example, the employee may require time to attend medical appointments or may need to use specific medical equipment during working hours that would be difficult to conceal.

Types of disclosure

Evans (2019) investigated the manner in which those who developed invisible illnesses (through accident, injury, or illness) disclosed their condition, to friends, colleagues, and supervisors and suggests that three forms of disclosure are used: confessional, pragmatic, and validating. Confessional disclosure occurs when a person uses disability to explain poor performance. For example, those adopting a confessional approach to disclosure may describe "fessing up" or "being caught". As described by one person, "I did kinda sit down with my manager … and just say, 'Hey, I'm having this issue, and, you know, I apologize if I'm not doing as well, but here's what's going on'" (Evans, 2019, p. 734). This form of disclosure may exacerbate existing internalized stigma, contributing to feelings of shame or guilt.

Pragmatic disclosure is typically fact-based and used to obtain support or accommodations. Needs are clearly expressed and the expectations of the employer or colleague are carefully managed. As one person described their pragmatic disclosure, "I needed to let these people who count on me at a distance to work my ass off know that maybe I'm not going to … I needed to communicate in order to regulate the amount of demand that my fellow [colleagues] were making of me" (Evans, 2019, p. 737). Validating forms of disclosure frame disability as a legitimate identity, with people disclosing in order to demonstrate that their difference is legitimate or authentic. This form of disclosure allows those with invisible disabilities to identify allies, support others, or recognize those who are not supportive. One person reported, "I want them to see me holistically. I want them to see my passion and hear a little bit of my story, and I don't ever wanna cut something out of my life in my identity" (Evans, 2019, p. 741).

There are other important aspects of the disclosure process. For example, people who decide to disclose an invisible condition may engage in protective disclosing or spontaneous disclosing (Charmaz, 1991). Protective disclosing aims to control when, how, and what people disclose about their condition and involves careful planning and preparation. In contrast, spontaneous disclosure is typically associated with shock or new information (e.g. revealing a new diagnosis to colleagues before they have fully processed the information themselves). In addition, people with disabilities may also engage in signalling, such as dropping hints or discussing subjects that are relevant to the disabled identity, which encourage others to 'read between the lines' (Woods, 1994). In addition, after self-disclosure, those who have revealed a disability may engage in a process of normalizing – that is, revealing the stigmatized identity but then attempting to minimize differences between that and a "normal" identity. For example, a person may seek to minimize the severity of symptoms or frequency of symptom flares.

Non-disclosure and passing

Based on their level of disclosure, Ragins (2008) identifies three potential identity states. These are identity denial, identity integration, and identity disconnect. Those with identity denial are aware of their stigmatized status but conceal this across both work and non-work settings. Identity denial provides little opportunity to access practical or social support. Identity integration involves full disclosure in both work and non-work contexts. Identity integration removes the risk that a person will be "outed" more widely after disclosure to specific individuals. Indeed, some people may lose control of the disclosure process; for example, after confiding in one colleague the subject may become "office gossip". This outing may be intentional or it may be an unintended consequence of not realizing that some people know and others do not. Alternatively, the person who outs their colleague may not understand the importance of the information they reveal and the consequences of this for the stigmatized individual.

Identity disconnect occurs when a person discloses a stigmatizing identity to varying degrees across work and non-work contexts. As described by one of my interviewees: "*I disclosed to my Head of School, who's been pretty supportive about the whole thing. I think his approach is a 'whatever, what can we do for you?' It hasn't been necessary to go any higher up management than that, but I would start to feel wary at that point anyway. And quite a few of my colleagues are also friends. So I've been quite happy to tell them but I haven't gone broadcasting it*" (Academic 3). Presentation of different identities in different domains can lead to anxiety and stress. Those who choose to partially disclose across domains may find it difficult to monitor who knows their stigmatized identity and the extent to which they have detailed information about it (e.g. symptom severity). This highlights the incidence and impact of covering a disability. Solis (2006) describes the process of concealing his emotions: "there are varied and often contradictory emotions that accompany living with multiple disabilities. For instance, in public I always strive to present a cheerful and positive demeanor, whereas in private I frequently experience frustration, anxiety, anger, and fear stemming from the fact that my body literally collapses from exhaustion" (p. 146).

Passing refers to "a cultural performance whereby one member of a defined social group masquerades as another in order to enjoy the privileges afforded to the dominant group" (Leary, 1999, p. 85). In this manner, a person with an invisible disability may be incorrectly categorized as a person without a devalued (i.e. disabled) identity. Stigmatized individuals may use a range of tactics in order to pass, including fabrication, concealment, and discretion (Herek, 1996). Fabrication involves deliberately providing false information about the self to others, concealment is actively preventing people from obtaining information about oneself, whilst discretion involves attempts to avoid questions relating to the stigmatized identity (Herek, 1996). Of course, whilst those with invisible disabilities may pass as non-disabled in order to avoid prejudice and discrimination, the process of passing can be a source of significant emotional stress which requires considerable time and energy and can contribute to poor mental and physical health (La Monica, 2013). Passing may also contribute to isolation and a fragmentation of the self (e.g. between work and non-work domains).

Responses to disclosure

It is important to acknowledge that disclosure does not necessarily lead to acceptance by others or understanding of the condition. As described by one interviewee: *"We've got quite a small teaching team for our subject area, there's only [number] of us and everybody knows ... they all know. I don't think they necessarily appreciate on a day-to-day basis, the impact that it has or when I'm having a good day or a bad day"* (Academic 1). Faculty described a range of responses to disclosure including negative responses and mistreatment. For example, *"I disclosed to the man I spoke to that I had been self-harming that day. And he said, 'Oh, um you're fine to be in work'. Basically, I was like, 'Wow' [academic laughs]. So that was just really, really substandard and very not supportive. And I was like, 'Did you hear what I just said to you?' So because I was really distressed, I was just like, I can't, there's nothing I can say. So I've actually kind of been really mistreated by, by management and by occupational health, that's kind of abusive from both of those people"* (Academic 4).

In particular, colleagues who are not disabled often fail to appreciate the importance of workplace accommodations or perceive these as an unfair advantage. As recalled by another interviewee: *"One of them would often,* almost every time, one of them would often say, 'I'd love to take a day a week off'. And it's like, 'you know you can ask for that. You can work four days a week, you've actually got a legal right to request you know, flexible and part-time working, you can literally go right now and decide you want less money. Oh no you prefer money, me too.' And a very sort of aggressive, almost ... the sense that I was taking holiday a lot. But I'm not, I'm unconscious. I'm not unconscious, I'm barely conscious in bed for the day most times. So it's not like I'm having a fun day off. I'm mostly trying to get to the point where my brain works enough to work again while often answering emails or doing marking or doing other things that are lower-level cognition"* (Academic 11).

It is important that those listening to a disclosure respond with empathy and acceptance rather than doubt, invasiveness, or paternalistic pity. It is also important to avoid comparisons that, whilst often intended to demonstrate shared experience and solidarity, serve to undermine the impact of disability. This may be especially important for symptoms such as fatigue that are often inappropriately compared to routine tiredness. One interviewee explained: *"It's kind of like when people go, 'Oh, I'm anxious'. And they go, 'Yeah, well, everyone's worried'. That's not what I'm saying, though, is it. You could have said, 'What are you anxious about? What can I help you with?' Fair enough, we are all anxious, but that's just closed down my conversation. And I feel like there's a lot, a lot of people who still do that. And they don't say, 'Well, could you explain that to me'. There's a time for you to discuss your issues and there's a time for me to discuss mine. It's not a competition"* (Academic 6).

Academics reported that their own openness often encouraged others to disclose. As described by another of my interviewees: *"The interesting one is how suddenly, or not suddenly but how once you share how many people share back, and quite personal stories that probably they might have not said to anyone else. But somehow by opening up that little door people share back and open up something from their side as well. That's been quite interesting, actually"* (Academic 9). The shared experience of disability was also discussed in relation to students. Faculty often commented that they revealed their condition in response to a student's self-disclosure or that they disclosed in order to provide a safe space for student disclosure. For example, *"I have said to students, 'I've had anxiety, depression forever, so if you need to talk about mental health, literally, nothing scares me. Because I've been there, I am there, it's okay'. I've said that to people in classes, I've said that to personal tutees individually. I've been like, 'Look, it's safe for you to talk about mental health'"* (Academic 4).

Goffman (1963) adopts the term 'wise' to refer to non-stigmatized people who have some insight into the experiences of those who are stigmatized and are sympathetic to it. Wise individuals may protect or insulate the disabled person from unwelcome or uncomfortable interactions with others. Non-stigmatized allies may promote acceptance and inclusion, such as when confronting discrimination or reacting positively to the disclosure of invisible disability (Law et al., 2011; Rasinski & Czopp, 2010), which can reduce the burden on disabled faculty. Indeed, allies have supported the inclusion of ethnic minority, sexual minority, and female employees (e.g. Ballard et al., 2008; Reason et al., 2005).

Supportive colleagues with positive responses to disclosure are especially important given the isolation and exclusion often experienced by people with disabilities. Whilst social isolation is important in any context, it may be particularly detrimental in the academic environment where people are often dependent on collaborative relationships for professional activities (e.g. invited presentations) and career progression (Ragins, 2008). Supportive allies can also engage in advocacy, extending beyond a passive acceptance of the stigmatized group to active attempts to change the organization or environment. It is important to emphasize that non-disabled academics can and should become allies who challenge academic ableism even if a colleague has not personally disclosed a disability. This reduces the pressure on disabled faculty to self-advocate or disclose.

For example, social events that attempt to foster positive working relationships often exclude disabled members of staff. Disabled staff may, therefore, feel under pressure to reveal their disability in order to provide a "valid" excuse for non-engagement or fear being perceived as unfriendly or socially distant. As described by one of my interviewees: *"School events will be a five aside football match ... they just don't think when they put these things on. And then you're like, well, that's great, no it's alright, thanks. Or we're gonna have a Thursday lunchtime 10k run. And I'm like, No, we're not. It's that ablest approach. It's not intentional whatsoever, but because the majority of the staff, you know they're in their 30s, or 40s, and they're active in sports with no health conditions, they're just not aware"* (Academic 1). Of course, the way in which planned events are discussed and advertised is also important. The suggestion that "we can't do that because of equality and diversity/disability", etc. is unfair and likely to make disabled members of staff feel uncomfortable. The emphasis should be on wanting to be inclusive and not on blaming disabled staff for being unable to host specific activities.

Summary

Whilst disability-oriented research often focuses on visible conditions (e.g. wheelchair users), a significant number of disabled people have conditions that are not immediately apparent to others. Those with invisible conditions must repeatedly decide whether to disclose. Those who choose to disclose have also to consider the amount and type of information to be revealed and the people who will have access to this information. Self-disclosure has the potential for both positive (e.g. access to workplace accommodations) and negative (e.g. discrimination) consequences. It is, therefore, essential that those responding to self-disclosure do so with sensitivity and respect.

Status and reputation

Reputation management forms an important part of academia. For example, faculty often establish a social media presence to publicize their research and contribute to scholarly debate. Those wishing to conceal disability, perhaps concerned that this will negatively impact on their "professional image", may find it difficult to manage long-term health conditions. For example, when faced with "away days" and extended meetings it could be difficult for someone to check and manage insulin levels, take medication, move around to ease pain and help mobility, etc. As explained by one academic I interviewed: *"There's a lot of pressure to seem clever and switched on, interesting and awake, and be constantly making those connections with other people. You know, that kind of casual networking stuff. I don't want people to see me when I am really cognitively burned out. I don't want to have that interaction. Because I want to be, especially because I'm very early career, I want the impression that I leave, I need the impression that I leave, to be somebody who's interesting, switched on here and ready for it"* (Academic 12).

Job security may also be important when considering whether to disclose a disability or chronic illness. As commented by one disabled academic, "[Y]ou don't want to rock the boat too much if you don't have tenure … I mean they're not supposed to ever fire you because you have a disability; however, in the real world, you know, would you be granted tenure, would that be held against you" (Stone et al., 2013, p. 164). As a consequence, faculty are more confident disclosing when they have reached a level of professional success or security. For example, one interviewee explained: *"I was very shy, in my early career of saying I was dyslexic. In fact, when I applied to do a PG Cert, I didn't declare it at all, because I thought there's no way they will let me on the course if they know I'm dyslexic. Only through my doctorate experience, have I almost inverted commas 'come out' as being dyslexic. And since then, I shout it from the rooftops and challenge people"* (Academic 2), The same academic stated: *"It's only really since my doctorate have I spoken up, because I think I've had the legitimacy to go, you know, yes, I'm a doctor now. So deal with it. And yes, I'm a professor now deal with that"* (Academic 2).

5 Experiences of disabled academics

Personal accounts provide an especially valuable insight into the issues faced by disabled academics, both with respect to the specific condition experienced and the institutional ableism encountered. I focus here, therefore, on personal experiences of disability within higher education. The chapter is informed both by existing research literature and a series of individual interviews that I conducted with higher education faculty. In addition to a number of shared experiences identified by disabled academics (e.g. the decision to disclose), there are, of course, issues specific to particular conditions. I highlight the specific challenges experienced by academics with autism, dyslexia, mental health conditions, musculoskeletal disorders, and energy-limiting conditions.

Identity, stigma, and disclosure

All of my interviewees met the formal criteria for disability. There was, however, a general reluctance to personally identify as disabled. For some academics, this reflected a fear that they were not 'disabled enough'. For others, their condition was perceived as a strength rather than a weakness and did not fit the traditional narrative of 'dis-ability'. Willingness to identify as disabled had important consequences for both the individual academic and wider disabled community. On an individual level, those who did not identify as disabled were less likely to formally declare a disability or seek support. As a result, the data available on disability within higher education is inaccurate and fails to capture the presence of disabled faculty or represent the disabled academic community. As summarized by one of my interviewees: "*It's underreported, but it's also that we don't have the language or the systems to report on it. Because this word, this phrase, 'Do you consider yourself disabled?' No, I don't. But unless I tick it, I won't appear in any data. And that ... that is a problem*" (Academic 2).

Faculty were also reluctant to disclose a disability for fear of discrimination (see also Chapters 2 and 4). For example, one interviewee commented: "*Often now on forms, I'll be 50-50. Like, sometimes I'll tick 'no' and sometimes I'll tick 'yes'. Just depending on what I'm filling the form in for and what I think the implications might be of me disclosing stuff. So I'm quite guarded about it. Not through shame, which I think is what I was feeling before, but through just political awareness, I'll put it that way*" (Academic 4). Indeed, many academics reported negative reactions from their colleagues or were aware that other disabled faculty had been mistreated. One interviewee described the perspective taken by colleagues as follows: "*If you've got that then how can you be an academic? How can you have cognitive dysfunction and be a high-flying academic, your brain doesn't work? No, it doesn't work in certain areas, so it's got nothing to do with my intelligence. And I've got all the documentation, part of the reason I went through the cognitive testing was to show how high functioning I am in the majority of areas, so it's not affecting my intelligence. I'm not teaching the students all gobbledegook because my head's messed up, which is what somebody said to me*" (Academic 1) (see also Chapter 6).

The academic environment

Management of health conditions was made more problematic by the intensification of academic workloads. As one interviewee explained: "*One of my first line managers was really good because he said, 'Okay, we'll have like a traffic light system, where if you think that you're going to start getting into a flare type situation, then let me know it's that sort of amber level because we can look at doing something and working with you so it doesn't get worse and progresses into that red'. That was in the good old days, when there was actually time to be able to do this and without the additional work pressures that have been imposed. Another one of the things is that the workload has just ramped up over the last four or five years. And the role, as you probably appreciate, is just totally different to what it was when I went into it*" (Academic 1). Organizational approaches to illness were perceived to be especially challenging. As another interviewee explained: "*You know, sometimes you do just need a day off sick because your brain is not working and there's nothing you can do about it. And then to integrate that into a disciplinary process is just so demoralizing. You'd probably have more academics with these conditions if you didn't chase them all out*" (Academic 11).

Whilst some academics believed that there was no opportunity for them to progress within academia (unless there was substantial structural and cultural change), others were focused on challenging ableism and developing a more inclusive environment. These approaches were not necessarily mutually exclusive, with a range of complex emotions experienced. As one of my interviewees described: "*Some of it, I would say, you just have to suck it up. Because there's not much you can do about it. And there's no point trying to get too bothered about things you can't control. And yet, at the same time, the bit that shows that you're not really reconciled to it, is that I think fairly frequently about leaving. You know, thinking this isn't a job in which people like me can survive or perform well. Even though I think all things being equal, I have the capability to do it, I don't have the capacity to do all the add on stuff. And so I do think about those kinds of things, you know, when I think I'm just gonna have to go, because there isn't room for me in a role like this. And then at other times, I allow some of that righteous indignation to make me gird my loins and fight back, you know, because it's so ablest it's untrue. Unless you are an all-singing, all-dancing performer, who is absolutely outstanding, then there's no space for you. And it shouldn't be like that. It's like that structurally, it's like that systemically. So I suppose I sort of oscillate between the two, really, I will take up my space here, and I will try to make a change and I've had enough of this, I think I'll just give up, get out*" (Academic 10).

Autism

The number of autistic people entering higher education, both students and faculty, has increased. This reflects improved diagnosis of autism and reporting procedures and widening participation initiatives. Characteristics of autism vary widely, though social and communicative challenges are commonly experienced and autistic people are often sensitive to change (APA, 2013). Common co-morbid conditions include anxiety and depression (Boyd et al., 2011). Though a considerable body of autism-oriented research is available, this typically focuses on autism in children, with relatively few studies addressing autism in older adolescents or adults. As a consequence, there is relatively little research investigating the experiences of higher education students or faculty who are autistic (Gelbar et al., 2015).

Students and faculty may not have received an official autism diagnosis or be reluctant to disclose. As a consequence, higher education institutions are often unaware that there are autistic students or faculty who require support (White et al., 2011). Common challenges include the lack of structure to higher education (compared with previous education) and group work. One student discussed the difficulties associated with group work and in particular self-monitoring of performance with peers: "That causes extra stress, and is yet another energy cost that you have to invest to perform well in a group project. You need to find an answer to the set problem, but you also have to make sure you are functioning in a group properly" (van Hees et al., 2015, p. 1679).

The issues experienced by students and the challenges to be addressed do, of course, vary. For example, Anderson (2018) explored the experiences of autistic students using university libraries and library resources. Whilst some students reported frustration that the library did not provide the quiet environment expected (and therefore experienced overstimulation), others found it difficult to adjust to library social norms (e.g. lowered voices). Private study rooms or cubicles were especially valued, as these afforded some protection from both noise and other distractions, suggesting that open plan offices or large conferences may be problematic for autistic acdemics. Indeed, one academic I interviewed described the stress associated with unwanted noise and requests for workplace accommodations: "*I said that I was finding noise in the building where I was working to be a stressor. And there was ... it happened quite quickly after that point that my office was moved. And so, I have an office in a quieter part of the department. And I think disclosing might have helped with that. Because I think it made it clearer to my Head of School that unwanted noise wasn't just annoying, because I had mentioned it before.*

And it was. 'We'll look into it if we can', but as soon as I said, it's a stressor to me and it interacts with this condition, then something happened fairly quickly" (Academic 3).

Cai and Richdale (2016) investigated the experiences of autistic college and university students via focus groups with students and their family members. Whilst family members reported that both educational and social support were poor, students reported that they were educationally but not socially supported. Whilst the reasonable adjustments made by universities to support autistic students may include practical measures such as a mentor who provides support with organizational skills, it may be more difficult to address other issues (such as societal acceptance) that also impact on experiences of higher education. These same societal attitudes may also have a substantial impact on colleagues' behaviour towards autistic peers (e.g. willingness to engage in interaction or interpretation of behaviour) and research addressing this issue is urgently required.

Academic progression is influenced, to a considerable extent, by social interactions. For example, discussions at a conference may lead to research collaboration, and informal "water cooler" discussions may lead to an invitation to join a faculty committee. Such interactions may be more challenging or stressful for autistic colleagues. The move to remote working during the COVID-19 pandemic may, however, have reduced the number or impact of these interactions. As one interviewee explained: "*It's reduced all of those funny little social interactions that I find hard. So I don't run into somebody and have to be in social mode when I wasn't expecting it. And I really appreciate that. And there's been lots of stuff written about how Zoom and so on is exhausting for people because they don't have 'the normal' cues that help them with the back and forth and people are talking over each other a lot more. And everyone's finding it stressful. And I went 'Oh, right. So everybody is now experiencing social interactions the way that I do'*" (Academic 3).

For some faculty and students, the discipline itself may present issues of representation and inclusion. For example, one student stated:

> "My psychology test literally had 'autistics don't use words like think or feel' as a 'correct answer' on the test ... when I emailed my professor research showing this isn't in fact true, she ignored me ... and now is really passive aggressive with me and tries to intimidate me in class" (Gelbar et al., 2015, p. 49).

Another commented: "The way that psychology classes and textbooks describe autism is often insulting, and presented entirely from a neurotypical point of view. Any classroom discussion of autism should include autistic perspectives, and be mindful of the idea of neurodiversity" (Sarrett, 2018, p. 686). Similar issues may, of course, be experienced by academics delivering or assessing such content.

Strengths rather than deficits

Though few studies have investigated the experiences of autistic academics, more information is available addressing the experiences of faculty working with autistic students (Gobbo & Shmulsky, 2014). For example, faculty have reported that autistic students may be less likely to notice non-verbal social cues (e.g. indicating that the focus of a task has changed), may not follow traditional physical boundaries (e.g. standing too close), and are more likely to experience anxiety. However, faculty have also recognized the academic strengths associated with autism, including passion for the subject area and a desire to obtain accurate information about the subject. One professor commented:

> "The students certainly changed my stereotype of autistic people. I had always thought of them as somewhat remote, un-related, un-responsive, etc. The two I had this semester were extremely friendly and related, to me and the other students. One is so connected that he has been hired as a freshman orientation leader. He will do a fine job" (McKeon et al., 2013, p. 356).

Indeed, there is increasing recognition of the strengths (rather than deficits) associated with autism, both within education and wider society. For example, autistic students identify a number of benefits of the condition such as focus and dedication, observational skills, and impartiality (van Hees et al., 2015). Though these are more commonly discussed in relation to students, these strengths also extend to autistic faculty. Robertson and Ne'eman (2008) highlight the importance of addressing the wider campus community culture. They argue that the "spirit of autistic acceptance on campus should focus on embracing autistic college students' diverse gifts, talents, and abilities, while acknowledging and respecting their autonomy, individuality, and rights and responsibilities" (p. 10). They further state that higher education institutions "must strive to empower autistic college students and foster their personal growth, rather than seeking to normalize them" (p. 10).

Dyslexia

A substantial body of research has documented the challenges faced by dyslexic students. For example, dyslexic students report a lack of information about entering higher education (Madriaga, 2007), are less likely to complete their higher education programme of study, and obtain a lower classification of degree than non-dyslexic students (Richardson & Wydell, 2003). Negative experiences are also reported by students during their professional or clinical training. Investigating the clinical experiences of student nurses, Morris and Turnbull (2006) report that disclosure of their dyslexia was an issue for all students interviewed. Whilst some participants disclosed in order to receive accommodations, others chose not to disclose and feared that they would be "talked about" or allocated inferior duties.

One student nurse explained, "I'd get the rubbish jobs, any HCA jobs, when they should be taking you through the practice of the core nursing staff" (Morris & Turnbull, 2006, p. 241). Another stated: "When they find out they withdraw from you and make out you're not on the same level … they try to rubbish you and make you feel you've got nothing in your brain" (Morris & Turnbull, 2007, p. 38). Indeed, the disclosure process was perceived to be threatening and stressful. A further student nurse commented: "No one knows about it – I can't bring myself to say it. I hated to be labelled as having it [dyslexia]. I just can't and I hate it" (Morris & Turnbull, 2006, p. 242). These concerns may remain after professional qualification. For example, one qualified medical practitioner commented: "Dyslexia is actually quite a big thing. And there's obviously a lot of stigma behind it ... Because it's so stigmatising ... I think people will, erm, view me in a different light for it" (Shaw & Anderson, 2017, p. 3). Self-doubt was also apparent, with the same practitioner reporting, "I felt like my BRAIN wasn't as good as other people's brains" (Shaw & Anderson, 2017, p. 5).

For many academics, their first instinct may be to reassure students and highlight the benefits of self-disclosure (i.e. access to accommodations and support). Indeed, Ryder and Norwich (2019) report that lecturers in British universities typically display positive attitudes towards dyslexic students and related accommodations. This may not, however, reflect the attitudes or behaviour of all educators. Evans (2014) investigated the attitudes of nursing lecturers towards dyslexic student nurses. Lecturers prioritized "getting the work done" and expressed concerns about their students' ability to cope with the demands of the nursing role on placement or in post qualification practice. One lecturer stated that some

> "students are severely dyslexic and they need a reader and that causes [a] huge amount of problems because in this profession you have to be honest, if they can't read the instruction in a chart, if they can't tell the difference between duphalac and digoxin you've got patient safety issues" (p. e44).

It is, therefore, essential to ensure that those who do disclose are not stigmatized or disadvantaged.

Dyslexic teachers and academics

> I have been actively trying to reframe what it means to be dyslexic. Since I started teaching I have argued that being dyslexic helps me teach students who find it difficult to learn or write because I find some things difficult and have many 'tactics' to overcome such difficulties. (Skinner, 2011, p. 132)

In contrast to the student-oriented research, there is a paucity of information about the experience of dyslexic educators. Similar to dyslexic students, academics may be reluctant to disclose their dyslexia to employers and adopt a range of strategies to minimize the visibility or impact of the dyslexia, such as working longer hours. Indeed, dyslexic newly qualified and trainee teachers report fearing being "found out" by their colleagues (Riddick, 2003). In part, these anxieties may reflect the negative and humiliating early experiences of formal education reported by dyslexic postgraduates and academics (Collinson & Penketh, 2010). To some extent, academia offered these individuals an opportunity to address these early experiences. As the authors comment, "the ability to perform well academically as graduate and postgraduate students was offered as a way of laying claim to an elite learner identity that others had suggested would remain inaccessible" (Collinson & Penketh, 2010, p. 15).

For dyslexic faculty, the traditional emphasis on written academic work is a substantial barrier to progression. As one of my interviewees explained: "*I still have issues about the fact that there's not a lot of neurodiversity in higher education. The norm is still read-write, conventions still read-write. The reason I'm a Professor of Learning and Teaching is the fact that I would never have got a traditional research professorship because I hate writing for academic publication. I find the whole process scary, off-putting, soul destroying because of the kind of views and attitudes towards this kind of quite a brutal way of providing feedback, if you write an article. So I've often chosen, I can present till the cows come home. I do conferences, international conferences, put me in front of thousands of people, don't bat an eyelid. Ask me to submit to a journal and I go back to a sort of frightened 15-year-old who's had to go in, 16-year-old have to go to do a GCSE exam, you know. And that has had a real impact on me in one sense. But also, in another sense I've kind of owned my career. And I've challenged them, I've done things differently, and I now encourage other people to do things differently*" (Academic 2).

Teachers with dyslexia report resilience and a range of coping strategies such as task-focused strategies (e.g. visualization or additional preparation), personalizing work contexts (e.g. incorporating their strengths into teaching practice), engaging with social support networks (e.g. collaborative work), and developing self-esteem and self-efficacy (Burns et al., 2013). Of course, such strategies may be less feasible for some lecturers. For example, Skinner (2011) describes how her role as a mother limited the strategies used to overcome her dyslexia (i.e. additional time that could be spent on tasks). Despite this, dyslexia appeared to provide some benefits, such as allowing her to understand the experience of existing on the margins in higher education.

Though typical of the disability field, descriptions of dyslexia usually focus on deficits and it is important to recognize the strengths associated with dyslexia. One interviewee reported: "*I didn't know till I had my dyslexia support, my full education psychologist's report, and that really helped me understand ME better. That helped just having some strengths, because perhaps until I'd had that done, all the weaknesses were pointed out to me, but not the strengths. So spatial awareness is a strength, verbalizing arguments is a strength. I kind of think, okay I can then say to somebody, this is what you need to do with me, give me problems to solve, give me things to work on, give me things that's creative, and I'll be effective*" (Academic 2). She felt it important to acknowledge and publicize these strengths: "*I am in a reasonably senior position that I can now start to make a bit more of a difference. So people don't understand the differences of dyslexia and don't understand the benefits. And I always try to say the benefits as well*" (Academic 2)

Indeed, teachers and trainee teachers often report that the advantages of being dyslexic outweigh the disadvantages. For example, dyslexia promotes creativity, empathy, and an understanding of student difficulties (Miller, 2011;

Riddick, 2003). One lecturer stated: "I think that because I am dyslexic I am able to see traits in others and openly share my diagnosis to demonstrate to students that it does not mean that they are not clever not that they won't achieve" (Ryder & Norwich, 2019, p. 164). In this manner, dyslexic educators can provide important role models. As stated by one dyslexic trainee teacher: "Explaining to the children that everyone needs some help sometimes was easier than I initially thought. It was also inspiring at times, for all the children that felt that they often needed help" (Glazzard & Dale, 2013, p. 30). To some extent, this may be an important motivation for the academics themselves. Robinson (2015) states: "Many times I wanted to quit but could not. My academic journey has never been about me. My goal is to inspire other students with dyslexia not to listen to educators who discourage them from achieving their goals. Ultimately, it is about them succeeding and graduating" (p. 42).

Mental health conditions

Mental health is a widespread and increasingly acknowledged concern. A significant proportion of the population experience some form of mental distress and academia is no exception. Conditions such as anxiety and depression impact on a substantial number of academics and students (Woolston, 2018); indeed, some aspects of academia may actively contribute to the incidence and experience of mental health conditions. Factors contributing to poor mental health in faculty include high teaching loads, a culture of extreme competitiveness, and a focus on long working hours (Costa et al., 2005; Rawlins, 2019). Indeed, the pressure to "keep up" or exceed the productivity of colleagues increases stress, creates tension between work and home life, and provides little time for self-care or maintaining the social support networks that are so important for our mental and physical health.

During one interview, the academic stated: "*I've always had anxiety and some form of depression on and off, and it's very much, all of it is exacerbated hugely by work*" (Academic 4). These issues appear to be embedded within higher education. The same interviewee commented further: "*It's almost like a badge people wear. Being exhausted and being stressed is like a kind of source of ... people wave it like a flag. So sometimes when you say, 'Oh, you know, my mental health is really bad'. And then people will say, 'well, isn't, isn't everyone's', it's just how it is in this culture. So you get constantly dismissed, and you're not visible as somebody with a mental health disability, because everyone is so stressed and so tired all the time, that you're not ... no one listens and no one takes it seriously, because that's just the badge that they wear, being exhausted and being hyper stressed*" (Academic 4).

In the United States, most faculty members are on non-tenure track contracts which typically provide fewer benefits and protection (Baldwin & Wawrzynski, 2011). Appointments may depend on student enrolments or other budgetary issues, leading to substantial uncertainty and stress. An inability to secure a permanent academic position is associated with anxiety and depression (Reevy & Deason, 2014). The academic culture that has arisen in response to increased student tuition fees may also impact on academic mental health. In particular, hostility targeted at faculty and a "consumer attitude" amongst students and their parents have increased, making academia a more challenging environment (Delucchi & Korgen, 2002). Female academics may be especially susceptible to such hostility (Sprague & Massoni, 2005). Similarly, contrapower harassment (i.e. student incivility, bullying, and sexual attention aimed at faculty) is also problematic (Lampman et al., 2009).

For faculty required to support students on residential field courses, the stress associated with responsibility for student safety, social anxiety, and limited opportunities to engage with normal coping mechanisms are particularly problematic. As stated by one academic: "Fieldtrips are very isolating. I find that kind of intense scrutiny – being under the gaze of students and colleagues – difficult to cope with. I just want to get away from them!" (Tucker & Horton, 2019, p. 90). For those who have not disclosed, considerable energy can be spent attempting to "pass" or shield themselves from significant stressors. For example, "Plenty of times I have 'hidden' away from the crowd, in the minibus, pub or (on residentials) in my hotel room. In the past, this has led to anxiety and awkwardness with colleagues (e.g., wondering why I wasn't answering my hotel door or mobile phone)" (Tucker & Horton, 2019, p. 90).

As discussed throughout this book, those disclosing disabilities may experience stigma and discrimination. Mental health is particularly susceptible to misconceptions and stereotypes. As a consequence, academics may be especially cautious when disclosing a mental health condition to peers, employers, or students. Such disclosure can, however, be beneficial. England (2016) provides a personal reflection on her decision to disclose her mental health (bipolar) status. She describes the decision to disclose as both a personal and political issue. Disclosure was motivated by a desire to be open and authentic and a wish to reduce the stigma associated with mental health issues. England (2016) argues that as a result of the disclosure, she was able to focus her energies on productivity and wellbeing rather than attempts to conceal her bipolar status or anxiety that it would be discovered.

As with other conditions, mental health is typically discussed in terms of deficits or weakness. Despite this, people with mental health conditions may develop a particular strength or resilience. One of my interviewees stated that she had been *"to some really, really terrifying places and it kind of gives you less fear of other stuff. Like I've heard other people say this as well, like the whole pandemic and isolation is like ... people with depression, we were like born for this shit, you know. Like we've been through this before. All that anxiety that people are feeling. It's like, well, this is how I've been feeling my whole life, like that level of ... that level of just terror, like abject kind of fear about stuff. I've been living with that and managing that and managing my perceived risk of going outside. That's something I've been living with for, like, forever. And now people are newly having to deal with this idea that the outside world is a scary place. It's like welcome to the club ... So that is a strength,*

I think that I'm kind of quite well equipped to cope with distress, because I'm really used to feeling it" (Academic 4).

Autoethnographic accounts

Autoethnographic accounts can provide a particularly insightful description of the issues faced by academics experiencing mental distress. Campbell (2018) provides a powerful autoethnographic account of depression and anxiety in academia. She explains the difficulties associated with leave, sickness, and self-care in academia:

> "I took a week's holiday, and spent every day running over and over what I needed to do at work, and how I was going to do it. My brain never switched off. I woke up night after night at 2am like clockwork, checking my work emails on my mobile phone" (p. 236). On returning to work, she explained that "It only took one e-mail – one tiny message asking me to do something – to send me flying into the abyss. Goodbye ladder. Hello three months of sick leave" (Campbell, 2018, p. 236).

In one diary entry she explains how the experience of depression and anxiety impacted on her personal and professional identity. "I have let everyone down by being weak. My identity is revealed as a fraud ... I'm off sick. That's now part of my identity. The girl who couldn't cope. The girl who needs to be referred to Occupational Health. The weak one" (p. 236).

One reviewer cautioned Jago (2002) against publication of her autoethnography focused on depression within academia. Jago (2002) responded:

> "Perhaps publishing my story is just another way of slitting my wrists, trying to sabotage my career by boldly wearing the label of mental illness. The stigma associated with depression is very real; I have seen it in the eyes of friends, students, and colleagues ... But I don't think so. There's a difference between taking a razor blade to your arm and risking the social stigma of depression. I have spent a great deal of time examining my motives and I keep coming back to the same thought. If publishing this story does damage to my career, if some react by questioning my credibility as an author, my capacity to teach, my mental stability, then I believe that's the best reason to publish my story. Being depressed means that I (and others like me) face a particular set of emotional challenges that make my life extremely painful and difficult at times. Being depressed doesn't mean I am untrustworthy, incapable, or crazy" (pp. 753–754).

Musculoskeletal disorders

The term "musculoskeletal disorder" refers to a range of inflammatory and degenerative conditions such as osteoarthritis and rheumatoid arthritis, that affect the joints, ligaments, muscles, peripheral nerves, and blood vessels.

These conditions have a substantial impact on the individual's quality of life; people with musculoskeletal disorders such as arthritis often experience fatigue (Hewlett et al., 2011) and are at increased risk of depression (Matcham et al., 2013). The experience of musculoskeletal disorders in education has been considered, though research investigating these conditions in primary or secondary school teachers is more common than studies focusing on tertiary education. For example, musculoskeletal disorders have been reported in elementary school teachers (Cardoso et al., 2009), primary and secondary school teachers (Korkmaz et al., 2011), and special education teachers and teaching assistants (Cheng et al., 2016). Female teachers and those working longer hours or with a higher workload may be particularly susceptible (Erick & Smith, 2011).

The activities that are likely to increase the incidence of musculoskeletal disorders or exacerbate symptoms (such as reading, writing, and assessment) that typically involve adopting a "head down" posture in a seated position for lengthy periods of time are, however, common to teaching at all levels. In addition, specific disciplines such as dentistry (Harutunian et al., 2011) or music (Fjellman-Wiklund & Sundelin, 1998) may be especially vulnerable due to the emphasis on practical demonstrations and repetitive fine motor skills. For one academic whose condition was musculoskeletal in nature, the lockdown and COVID-19 pandemic provided an opportunity to reflect on the energy typically required to commute to campus and fulfil her duties. She recalled when the first lockdown was introduced: "*I remember thinking, 'thank God, I need a break, I absolutely need a break'. And looking back, knowing that I was going into teaching, I think what I needed was a physical break. That actually, the trudging around, in and out, the commute, the physical going round all the different buildings really was taking its toll. And then we've done since, since the lockdown, we've done one day [on campus]. And I did a lot less work than I would normally do in a day. I was doing about four hours of teaching. But in between times, I think I did another hour of emails in a sort of seven-hour day. And the rest was just sort of sitting there. I came home and I couldn't do anything that evening. I was on the sofa, like ah I'm a cabbage. And it really struck home to me ... now you get that when you're travelling anyway, you know, if you go to a conference, whatever you know that even the travel itself is exhausting. But just making me think of what was that doing to me, day in day out, that kind of level of physical activity*" (Academic 7).

In one personal account, Chouinard (1995) describes her experience as an academic with rheumatoid arthritis and how the condition impacts on her: "Rheumatoid arthritis is an activity-sensitive disease and each time I'd try to do a little more of my academic work my body would rebel with a flare-up," though the reactions of others were also important. She explains: "It hasn't been easy to deal with being a disabled 'other' academic. I still find myself cringing and looking away when people stare at me as I scoot across the University campus; reminding me that I am different" (p. 4). The process of obtaining accommodations such as accessible parking was particularly difficult. Chouinard (1995) recalls:

"I remember crying with frustration at work and at home because such a small request was being denied and because I was having to expend so much of my energy fighting to get adequate access to my workplace … I was simply too tired and sick to fight any more" (p. 5).

With regards to disclosure, musculoskeletal disorders may, to some extent, provide a "safer" forum to discuss disability with colleagues or students than other, more stigmatized conditions. One of my interviewees explained to me: *"It's also a really handy one to own in terms of talking about difference. So one of the things that I'd be passionate about, again, possibly due to my history, possibly due to upbringing, would be issues around equality, diversity, inclusion. And telling someone that you've been depressed in the past, especially if you're a [names specialism] is a bit of a risky ground. You know, there's some colleagues that you probably wouldn't want to go there. You can tell anyone that you've got arthritis, and that it'll just be 'Oh'. And even if that … because I'm so okay with it now, that even if they're a bit uncomfortable, I can ride it out, it's fine. But it's a really useful thing to be able to disclose to demonstrate difference and diversity and whatever. So in terms of talking to students about it, it's a really easy one to bring into the conversation, to say, 'Look, I've experienced this, and this is how it impacts me'. And then you open up those conversations with them about their differences and things that maybe they're ashamed of"* (Academic 7). Indeed, many interview accounts suggested a "hierarchy" of conditions where some would be disclosed and others hidden.

Energy-limiting conditions

For many disabled people, a lack of energy is a particularly prominent symptom. Such conditions include chronic fatigue syndrome and fibromyalgia. These conditions are also often associated with cognitive impairment such as difficulties with memory and concentration (Arnold et al., 2008; Shanks et al., 2013; Wearden & Appleby, 1996) typically referred to as 'brain fog'. These conditions are often unpredictable. Patients may report "flares" where symptoms are exacerbated or more acute. For example, stress, anxiety, and overwork are common causes of fibromyalgia flares (Vincent et al., 2016). One patient reported: "Stress I would say is my BIGGEST trigger. There are days that stress makes my life awful." And another: "I can induce a flare pretty easily if I work too much and don't rest enough. If I push myself too hard … I can expect a flare in the coming days" (Vincent et al., 2016, p. 465). There may not be an indication that a flare will occur. A third patient commented: "If you've ever had a flu sneak up on you after you went to sleep one night and you wake up with your entire body aching, you've got an inkling of what a flare is. It's not gradual" (pp. 465–466). Such unpredictability may make it difficult for people with these conditions to plan ahead and manage their time.

Some aspects of the academic role such as long working hours are particularly problematic for those with energy-limiting conditions. One of my interviewees explained: "*I'd be getting home at eight, nine o'clock at night. And then like I said, do that for kind of three, four days a week, then work from home one day, and just to kind of recover, kind of get all my sort of data in order, things like that. But then the toll would come. You have the weekend, you know. I'd end up sleeping kind of 15 hours a day, on Saturday and Sunday to recover from the kind of running around that I'd done for the study in the week*" (Academic 8).

Conferences are also problematic for those experiencing fatigue. For example: "*You go to the conference, and then there's a post conference poster session, and then there's the dinner, and it's sort of, you know, half past 10 at night, 11 o'clock at night. And I can't do it*" (Academic 5). These issues may not be easily addressed by part-time contracts. As this interviewee explained: "*The other problem with the hours creep in academia is that ... from every, everything that I've heard from everybody I've talked to, a part-time job is not part time. It's not part time, it just means that you will get paid less for doing almost the same amount of work. Which is horrendous. It's absolutely horrendous for anyone with the stamina impairment, because you have to be able to set boundaries and academia is almost philosophically opposed to the concept of people setting boundaries about their work.*"

It may be difficult for academics to accept that their role is limited by their energy levels. These issues are not, of course, restricted to conditions where fatigue is the primary symptom. For example, other academics experiencing fatigue report a number of emotions such as self-blame and guilt. During interview, one faculty member revealed that, "*I used to use it as a stick to beat myself with aaall the time. What I do with it now, I think I've accepted that I have some fairly stark limits on what I can do. And if I work evenings, and weekends, I will break*" (Academic 3). Another of my interviewees also acknowledged her situation: "*I've beaten myself up for years for the fact that I need lots of sleep ... for years, I've wanted to be able to come home, put the kids to bed and then do another three hours of work, because that's what academics do. Or get up, you know, all my friends over lock down ... academics who've got little ones are like, 'Oh, it's fine, I get up at five and do three hours, two hours before they wake up'. And I'm like, that's just not an option for me. And it's taken a long, long time for me to go well, I'm just a different kind of academic*" (Academic 7).

There is often a lack of understanding surrounding energy-limiting conditions, which impacts on both those who have a condition such as chronic fatigue syndrome and those whose wider symptom profile includes limited energy. For example, non-disabled colleagues may liken their own tiredness to the clinical fatigue experienced by disabled faculty. As one academic commented during interview: "*That's the classic one, isn't it? 'Oh, yeah. I'm exhausted as well. I've had a super busy day'. Yeah, I had that one yesterday. I was trying, I said, Look, no, I can't do this, because of the fatigue. 'Oh, yeah, I'm exhausted too. It's tiring, isn't it doing this online learning?' And I'm like,*

'Oh, you haven't got a clue'" (Academic 1). This rhetoric can make it hard for academics to recognize their own health issues. Another interviewee explained to me that *"I think everybody finds being an academic pretty tiring and so if you, if I said that I was feeling utterly wiped out, there's supposed to be 'Oh, that's normal'. And I don't think I realized that my levels of fatigue were that unhealthy, because I thought everybody was feeling like that"* (Academic 3).

Many energy-limiting conditions such as chronic fatigue syndrome and Lyme disease have a complicated history. For example, they have been contested within the medical profession and disparaged in the media as 'yuppie flu'. Those with misunderstood or contested conditions may be particularly reluctant to formally disclose their condition, and informal support may be especially important. One academic with Lyme disease described the value of this during our interview. She stated: *"My main research colleague, who was also a kind of senior research assistant, she had fibromyalgia. And so she'd actually been through a kind of a lot of the processes that I'd been through. And kind of gone through all of those, you know, people not really understanding or kind of thinking that you're exaggerating, or maybe, you know, making things up. So it was really nice to have someone there. If you are having a bad day, you could just look at them and say, 'I'm having a tough day today'. And they'd kind of almost know exactly how you felt. And likewise for her"* (Academic 8).

COVID-19

The experiences of disabled academics are, of course, influenced by a range of factors and individual disciplines may present specific challenges. For example, in Geography, Earth, and Environmental Sciences, fieldwork may be particularly problematic (Tucker & Horton, 2019). As stated by one academic: "I have never, either as staff or student, come home well from a residential fieldcourse" (Tucker & Horton, 2019, p. 84). Common issues impacting on academic wellbeing include the lack of access travelling to or when visiting field sites, physical exhaustion as a consequence of long working hours, stress for those responsible for student safety or teaching sessions, and social anxiety. The lack of rest or reflection time and distance from normal coping mechanisms such as social support appear to further exacerbate the difficulties of fieldwork. Despite these issues, there is often little support for academics engaging with fieldwork. As summarized by one academic, "I am seen as the problem, not the planning/practices!" (Tucker & Horton, 2019, p. 91).

Academics I spoke with emphasized the importance of COVID not just in terms of demonstrating opportunities to work at home, conduct remote interviews, etc., but also with respect to stigma and attitudes towards disability. One interviewee explained: *"I definitely think there's a stigma around these types of conditions. You know, like M.E. and you know, chronic fatigue syndrome or fibromyalgia and there's definitely a kind of like, 'well are they real'* kind of energy around them. But you know, having experience there, I can definitely say, 'Yes, they are real'. And I think it's interesting kind of reading everything about long COVID now, and this seems to be affecting thousands of people. And again, towards the start of the pandemic, it was a little bit, you know, 'they had it and they've gotten over COVID now, like, what's their problem?' And I think it's finally been recognized by the NHS as a genuine condition and something that needs funding and research and you know people need rehabilitation and help. And I hope this kind of feeds into the conditions I just mentioned, you know like Lyme, M.E. and things that ... You know, there's a lot of people out there who are just bundling along and maybe could do with some support. So hopefully, that's kind of a positive that comes out of COVID, is kind of awareness of these kind of post viral conditions that you know can be really limiting and you know really awful" (Academic 8).

Summary

Personal accounts convey the lived experiences of disabled academics including the challenges associated with specific conditions, the impact of the ableism experienced, and factors that exacerbate or weaken the impact of this ableism. It is important to recognize, however, that these personal accounts require a significant investment from disabled academics. For example, those contributing to equality, diversity, and inclusion events in order to promote an understanding of disability may not be compensated for their time. In addition, discussing personal experiences of disability may increase the risk of stigma and discrimination. It is important that the accounts provided by disabled academics (e.g. disclosure at training events and published autoethnographies) are valued by the academic community.

6 Perceptions of disabled academics and disability

Student perceptions of disabled academics may have implications for faculty progression (e.g. evaluations by the student body inform performance targets and promotion criteria). These perceptions may also influence faculty decisions to disclose a disability. Importantly, educators serve as role models with a considerable influence on student attitudes, beliefs, and behaviour. Therefore, the presence of disabled academics has important ramifications for the student body, particularly in relation to the experience of students who are themselves disabled. This chapter considers both disabled and non-disabled student perceptions of disability and the impact of disabled faculty presence and disclosure on the student experience. Specific issues (i.e. perceived "faking it" or malingering) that impact on attitudes and behaviour will also be addressed.

Student evaluations

As previously discussed in Chapters 1 and 2, people with disabilities are subject to stigma and discrimination. Students are not immune from the stereotyping and discrimination displayed by members of the general population and student bias can have important consequences for faculty members. Student evaluations are commonly used to assess individual academic, module, and programme performance. Indeed, student evaluations have increasingly become a mandatory rather than voluntary form of quality assurance (Shah & Nair, 2012), and are often used to inform academic progression, promotion, and redundancy decisions. It is argued that anonymous student evaluations allow students to provide feedback on their university experience without fear of negative repercussions, hence these surveys typically form a core component of the quality assurance process (Leckey & Neill, 2001). Despite the widespread adoption of these surveys, student evaluations appear to be subject to substantial bias.

A range of non-academic factors influence student perceptions (and ratings) of academic staff, such as age (Arbuckle & Williams, 2003) and physical attractiveness (Felton et al., 2008). In particular, researchers have documented the extent to which sex, sexual orientation, and cultural background influence student evaluations (e.g. Fan et al., 2019; Heffernan, 2021; Reid, 2010). For example, students may be more hostile to academics that do not meet gendered expectations, expecting greater pastoral care from female than male faculty (Sprague & Massoni, 2005). In one qualitative analysis of over 350,000 student survey responses, Adams et al. (2021) conclude that "there were gendered disparities in the evaluations of expertise and authority presented in the data, such that female-identified teachers were penalised for the same teaching practices for which male-identified teachers were rewarded" (p.18).

Bias expectations may also impact on the rating of disabled academics. As summarized by one of my female interviewees: *"If you're a male professor and you forget things, it's because you're a genius whose mind is on something else. And I think this is commonly believed and understood. And if you're a woman forgetting stuff, then 'Oh, is she menopausal' or 'Is she ditzy'. Or is she this and that, it's utterly different. And I think it's an amazing trick that has been pulled, that this sort of sketchiness or brain fog is actually seen as a sign of intellectual strength in men, I'm convinced of this. I know somebody who is also definitely autistic, but as a man he has never burned himself out worrying about social interactions, he just does them badly and then he moves on with his life. I could have had that ..."* (Academic 3).

There is, however, a paucity of research on student evaluations of disabled academics. In one hypothetical study, students reviewed the résumés of prospective (disabled or non-disabled) faculty members. Students reported being more positive towards disabled than non-disabled academics (Pfeiffer & Kassaye, 1991). Additional research is, of course, required to review student evaluations of actual disabled and non-disabled academics. Pfeiffer and Kassaye (1991) indicated disability status by describing the potential faculty member as a wheelchair user. Future research should include a wider range of disability types (e.g. sensory impairments, chronic health conditions). This research should also consider whether students believe that the disability has impacted on the learning and teaching practice (such as the availability of faculty members) and whether students are themselves disabled.

In addition to the numeric rating of academics, students may also provide qualitative comments in their evaluations. Survey responses (including the comments) are typically anonymous and the inclusion of abusive comments has been acknowledged. Abusive or inappropriate comments may be directed at the overall student experience or be directed at specific academic or professional services staff (Tucker, 2014). Research suggests that abusive comments are disproportionately targeted at faculty from marginalized groups and the proportion of abusive comments included in student evaluations appears to have increased (Tucker, 2014). It is important to note that these comments may not be restricted to formal student evaluations that are coordinated by the university. For example, sites such as 'RateMyProfessor' allow students to rate and review their faculty and this information is publicly available and inappropriate comments may also be posted to social networking sites (Jones et al., 2011).

Although there is clear evidence for bias impacting on student evaluations and the potential for abuse, few studies have considered the impact of this on faculty members. Research that has been conducted demonstrates that academic responses to student feedback can be emotional. As described by one academic: "At the time I was devastated ... I felt awful, absolutely awful ... Obviously people in the team were supportive ... they didn't make me feel it was all down to me, but that didn't stop me feeling that way at the time" (Arthur, 2009, p. 448). Feedback may also negatively influence academic practice. In particular, ratings appear to impact on academic self-efficacy and confidence that a positive relationship can be developed with the student cohort (Boswell, 2016; Kowai-Bell et al., 2012). Despite these issues, and the introduction of measures to address the systemic bias held by faculty (e.g. anonymous marking of student assessments), there have been few attempts to address prejudice within student cohorts or the impact of this on marginalized faculty.

As outlined, student evaluations can be subject to both conscious and unconscious bias. It is important to emphasize that this is not the only mechanism through which student bias can negatively impact on disabled academics. For example, during interview one academic described the experience of a colleague who had not disclosed dyslexia to her students: "*I have a colleague who has been bullied by students for her written English. It's one of the situations where at the moment she hasn't got the support, where she's doing online stuff, and some of her dyslexia comes out and students go, 'Oh, my God, call yourself an academic, and you can't even read and write'*" (Academic 2). These issues must be addressed in order to support disabled academics.

Academic role models

Prevailing stereotypes characterize disabled people as less competent than those without disabilities. As a consequence, the opportunities afforded to disabled people (e.g. challenging roles or professional courses) may be limited, with managers reluctant to provide those opportunities to disabled people. Repeated discrimination such as being assigned less challenging or responsible roles may impact on the development of skills and experience and subsequent career progression (Wilson-Kovacs et al., 2008). For people with congenital disabilities or disabled at an early age, the protective behaviours displayed by parents, siblings, and teachers may also limit experience. Internalization of competency-based stereotypes by disabled people may further lead to self-limiting behaviour such as a reluctance to apply for challenging roles.

The presence of disabled faculty challenges existing assumptions that disabled people cannot become academics. As described by one of my interviewees: "*There's sort of this vision of, 'Yes sure, there are disabled people at University – they're students'. Like they don't, we don't evaporate at age 21, like we're still here*" (Academic 11). Disabled academics may also act as role models and mentors, demonstrating to disabled students or less experienced disabled colleagues how to become successful in a particular context (Jones, 1997; Pritchard, 2010). Despite the importance of these role models for disabled people, academic literature and mentorship programmes have often focused on other role model types (e.g. female academics) rather than those with disabilities. For example, research indicates that female faculty with mentors report higher career satisfaction, more publications, and spending more time on high status research (Levinson et al., 1991).

Despite the paucity of disability-specific information, role models are likely to have an important impact on disabled students and staff. Role models perceived as similar may be especially beneficial, as they provide clear evidence that success is achievable and practical advice that is not available from others. These role models and mentors are especially important because people with disabilities may have reduced access to informal events that offer networking or mentoring opportunities such as academic conferences. As stated by one academic, "The impact that impairments have on academics' abilities to attend conferences, papers, meetings etc. has a knock on effect … When you go for promotion you have to cite distinguished referees to give you references, how can one do this if your opportunities for meeting other academics are constrained?" (Williams, 2011, p. 199). Similarly, one of my interviewees stated: *"Part of the problem is we're fucking exhausted, we don't have the time to build a support network for ourselves"* (Academic 11).

Support/guidance and inspiration/modelling are particularly important aspects of role modelling (Nauta & Kokaly, 2001). The most effective style of role model may, however, vary. Positive role models describe those who have achieved substantial success (e.g. received a prestigious award) and negative role models refer to those who have experienced misfortune (e.g. those who have experienced significant hardship or injury). Lockwood et al. (2002) argue that those motivated by positive outcomes (e.g. promotion) are most inspired by positive role models, whereas those motivated to avoid negative outcomes (e.g. avoiding failure) are most inspired by negative role models. Indeed, potential role models may not always inspire, especially if we compare our own (more modest) abilities to their substantive achievements. The impact of potential role models may depend on whether individuals believe that they are able to attain similar success. "Superstars" are inspiring when their success appears to be attainable (i.e. the individual believes that they have the time or ability to make a similar accomplishment). In contrast, superstars whose success is perceived as unattainable (i.e. the individual believes that they have missed their chance or do not have the required ability) may leave some self-deflated (Lockwood & Kunda, 1997).

There are, of course, a limited number of visible disabled faculty available to act as role models. Indeed, the lack of disabled role models in particular disciplines such as science and engineering has been noted (Alston & Hampton, 2000). Therefore, whilst it is important to acknowledge that the greater use of disabled role models is beneficial for students and less experienced academics, it may overburden the disabled educators available to adopt this role. More open disclosure from disabled faculty will increase the visibility of disabled role models and increase the range of impairments that are represented. As previously stated, the perceived similarity of an individual to the role model is important. There is also a "hierarchy of disability" with differing levels of social acceptance (Deal, 2006) and impairments impact on the academic role differently (see Chapter 5). Therefore, the presence of role models with a wide range of impairment types is especially important. It is understandable that some academics with disabilities are reluctant to adopt this role. For example, being critical of institutional policy, or advocating for the rights of disabled students and staff may be perceived as disruptive and there may be a fear of reprisals amongst disabled faculty adopting this role (Williams, 2011).

Disabled identity and disability pride

Disabled academic role models are also important for the development of a positive disabled identity. Societal representations of disability are often negative, with disabled people typically encouraged to hide, 'fix', or overcome their impairment. As members of a marginalized and stigmatized group, disabled people may attempt to improve their self-concept by concealing or minimizing the stigmatized identity in order to assimilate into the dominant (i.e. non-disabled) group. An alternative approach for disabled people wishing to improve their self-concept is to reject the stigma associated with disability, affirm a disabled identity, and explicitly align themselves with other members of the disabled community (Bogart, 2014). A disabled identity that encourages people with disabilities to take pride in their disabled status, engage in activism, and see the value in their disabled experience can be especially strengthened by engagement with members of the disabled community.

There are a number of advantages for those developing a strong disabled self-identity. For example, disability identity and disability self-concept predict greater satisfaction with life, even when taking into consideration other important factors such as self-esteem (Bogart, 2014). Indeed, people with disabilities share many experiences with those from other marginalized groups, such as stigma, discrimination, and unequal access to education, health care, and employment. Interventions intended to support other marginalized groups (e.g. LGBTQ Pride) may, therefore, provide important insights into the development of a positive disabled identity. Of course, a range of factors may impact on the development of a disabled identity. For example, people with congenital disabilities display a higher satisfaction with life and disability self-efficacy and hold a stronger disability identity. For people with acquired disability (developing in later life), their condition may represent a loss of the original identity. The development of a disabled identity may be especially difficult for individuals who stigmatized disabled people prior to their own impairment (Bogart, 2014).

Disabled self-efficacy is an important part of the disabled identity and influences the types of goals a person sets, their persistence, and overall success. It is important to emphasize that disabled self-efficacy is *not* a measure of the severity of the impairment, for example an individual may display high disability self-efficacy if they believe that they have the resources required to complete their desired activity. People with disabilities who are high on self-efficacy display better mental and physical health, including less pain, lower fatigue, and fewer depressive symptoms (Amtmann et al., 2012). They may also be more positive about their academic potential and performance. Therefore, practice and policy should aim to foster a disabled identity and disabled self-efficacy rather than attempt to 'normalize' disabled people (e.g. Bogart, 2014).

Non-disabled students

Non-disabled students also benefit from the presence and visibility of disabled academics. It is important to emphasize that it is not simply the opportunity to engage with disabled people that is beneficial. For example, if nursing students only encounter disabled people in their role as patient rather than as instructor, expert, or advocate, they may be *more* rather than *less* likely to perceive disabled people as vulnerable and dependent. Previous research indicates that whilst attitudes towards disability do not differ among students who have different levels of contact with disabled people, students with a disabled professor report more positive attitudes towards disability (Hayashi & May, 2011; Shannon et al., 2009). It is the position and status of disabled faculty that promotes an appreciation of equality, diversity, and inclusion issues. In this context, the disabled educator is clearly identified as a knowledgeable subject specialist and authority in their field, which directly challenges stereotyped assumptions that disabled people are less competent than their non-disabled peers (Clément-Guillotin et al., 2018).

In one case study with a disabled academic (quadriplegia mixed type cerebral palsy applied), Sheridan and Kotevski (2014) discuss the learning opportunities that are available to (business) students who would have otherwise received little formal exposure to disability studies. Some students appeared to be particularly reflective, for example: "I think working with someone with a disability has made me more aware of the challenges faced by people with a disability as well as breaking down a barrier between people with a disability and those without when considering people to work with" (Sheridan & Kotevski, 2014, p. 1167). Repeated contact may, however, be important as in initial encounters, some students may be discomforted to learn that their tutor is disabled. For example, one student commented: "I was surprised, purely because you don't expect people to have a disability and I have found that people often forewarn others of disabilities" (Sheridan & Kotevski, 2014, p. 1165).

Students educated by teachers with a disability, therefore, are exposed to both discipline-specific content and important information about disability, diversity, and inclusion (Pritchard, 2010). Indeed, the employment of disabled faculty may also signal the values of the higher education institution itself, directly demonstrating a commitment to equality, diversity, and inclusion (Sheridan & Kotevski, 2014). As stated by Anderson (2006), "Teachers with disabilities offer knowledge through their bodies and experiences that isn't usually part of the curriculum. Disabled teachers embody pedagogies of justice, interdependence, and respect for differences" (p. 368).

It is important that disabled faculty do not feel pressured to educate others about disability. For example, being "seen" and "othered" can be difficult for disabled academics, especially if they feel that this distracts from their subject specialism and status as an expert in their own discipline. There are, however, important advantages when disabled academics are visible. As stated by Pritchard (2010), "There may be 'discomfort' (for ourselves as teachers with disability and undoubtedly for others) associated with being visible, but the alternative only ensures continued exclusion from all levels of education and does nothing to challenge the exclusionary boundaries of the current dominant academic culture and ableist paradigm." (p. 47).

Academic experiences and disclosure

During interview, academics acknowledged the impact of their presence on others (both students and staff) who were also disabled. Indeed, one interviewee recalled the importance of a disabled role model in their own professional career: "*They talked about knowing someone within the hospital who was a [names role] in a wheelchair. And other medics and clinicians who had disabilities and it shouldn't be any kind of barrier. And so that was kind of like, 'Oh, okay, I'll see what I want to do' ... that stay in hospital really rewrote that story of this can get really bad, but you know what other people do this. And it's okay, to have those kind of ambitions ... I never met the woman. But just knowing she existed ... maybe she didn't exist, maybe they made her up to make me feel better. But just knowing she existed, at the time was really ... I don't know what the path would have been if I hadn't have had that. I just even now, you know, my God, 30 years, not quite 30 years, 25 years later, remember how powerful that was, just to hear. 'It's okay. People with disabilities, people in wheelchairs and people with things wrong with them, with chronic conditions, they do these kind of jobs in hospitals', was really incredibly powerful*" (Academic 7).

The academics I interviewed had typically discussed their impairment with students. This disclosure often occurred in response to a student disclosing their own condition. For example: "*I did have a master's student once talk to me about maybe having a future in academia. And they expressed a fear that it might not be for them. Because they had some long-standing mental health issues. And I hadn't been planning to disclose anything that day but I thought this was probably a good time to go, 'No, it will be hard. But I have some issues too and you know, quite a few of us do. So it doesn't necessarily mean that you don't have a place here'. And I think they found that quite helpful*" (Academic 3).

Academics also disclosed their own condition as a way to open discussions about equality, diversity, and inclusion, creating a safe and supportive space for student disclosure. For example: "*Before I started the lecture, I explained that I had post-traumatic stress disorder and suffered with depression and anxiety. And that I was telling them, because I knew some of them would suffer with some of ... some of those, and that if I can't disclose and be open about my own conditions, then how are we expecting society to change. And a few students emailed me. There were probably about a hundred students in the class, two students emailed me, some anonymous, some not, saying 'thank you for saying that, it made me feel a lot better'. One student in particular came to see me and said, 'You are the only other person I've ever known who suffered with post-traumatic stress disorder'. And we chatted, I told him some of the things, how it affects me, and he was so relieved, he was going [mimics wide arms and excited face] 'that, that happens with me as well'"* (Academic 5).

Discussing disclosure, another faculty member commented: *"I do think it's important you know so that students can see it. I mean, I'm supervising a project student this year, who's also a wheelchair user ... when she finds that she's got someone who understands her particular difficulties and her particular needs ... And I haven't done anything for her, you know, there's nothing, it's not like we go out and let's do wheelies together or anything. I haven't done anything different, it's just that she feels she's in a real safe space, to be able to talk about things to do with her disability, you know"* (Academic 10). Indeed, some academics reported that students specifically sought their supervision because of their condition. For example: *"I examine, supervise doctorates, and I have requests from people who are dyslexic to examine them, because they believe that I will see past what that might be hang-ups for other people"* (Academic 2).

'Faking it' and perceived malingering

A lot of research has focused on perceptions of people with disabilities or specific impairments. There is, however, another important issue that impacts on disabled people. Those with disabilities can be perceived as malingering (i.e. faking or exaggerating their condition in order to receive an unfair advantage or financial support). These issues negatively impact on the willingness of disabled people to disclose an impairment or seek support. Numerous forms of malingering have been discussed: pure malingering refers to false presentation of an impairment that does not exist, positive malingering refers to feigning symptoms that do not exist, and partial malingering refers to the conscious exaggeration of symptoms that do exist (Resnick, 1984). This simulation or exaggeration is believed to include the use of facial expressions, responses to standardized questionnaires, or reduced effort when completing physical assessments (Fishbain et al., 1999).

Of perhaps no surprise to the disabled community, research has often focused on the detection of malingering rather than the experience of being falsely suspected of simulating or exaggerating an impairment (Bianchini et al., 2005; Fishbain et al., 1999; Hopwood et al., 2010). Indeed, researchers have proposed a range of criteria that "should increase the clinician's index of suspicion that a claimant is malingering psychological distress after a traumatic incident" (Resnick, 1984, p. 35). These include: "The malingerer may assert an inability to work, but retain the capacity for recreation, such as enjoyment of theatre, television, or card games"; "The malingerer may try to avoid examination, unless it is required to receive some financial benefit"; and "The malingerer may have a history or previously incapacitating injuries and extensive absences from employment" (pp. 35–36). Standardized measures such as the Structured Inventory of Malingered Symptomology (SIMS) have also been developed to classify individuals as "honest" or "suspected malingerers" (Clegg et al., 2009).

Malingering and the detection of faked or exaggerated disability has also been investigated in an educational context. For example, Harrison et al. (2007) reported that "this study clearly demonstrated that the symptoms of ADHD are easily fabricated, and that simulators would be indistinguishable from those with true ADHD. In addition, students motivated to feign ADHD could easily perform poorly on tests of reading and processing speed, thus allowing them access to academic accommodations" (p. 577). It is perhaps not surprising, therefore, that disabled students are fearful that others perceive them to be lazy rather than impaired (Osborne, 2019). Comments from disabled students included: "I have never had a professor understand that when I miss classes it is because I am sick, and not because I'm just using my conditions as an excuse for laziness" (Osborne, 2019, p. 239).

The disabled academics I interviewed recognized the importance of this issue. When discussing their own impairments, they frequently made comments such as "*I think they think you're making it up*" (Academic 5) and "*They tend to think that you're making excuses*" (Academic 12). They felt that colleagues did not understand their impairment or the importance of the accommodations provided. They also wanted to prove their value as an employee before disclosing a disability. For example: "*I felt like it was important for her to know that I'm not the kind of person to make excuses or to fake being ill. So I wanted to make sure she knew that first, before I told her what my condition was*" (Academic 6). Disabled academics also recognized the impact that the burden of assessment and proof had on students. As stated by one faculty member: "*As soon as they've got a disability, they've got to go through this awful process of being assessed, of being judged. It's grounded in suspicion around the idea that maybe you're not really disabled, because we're not going to take your word for it, you have to go and prove it*" (Academic 10).

In part, misperceptions may reflect current conceptualizations of health and health assessment. As described by one of my interviewees: "*I think this is a problem with all kinds of variable disability, to be honest. It's just not a concept that people have in our culture. We used to have this sort of concept I might add but we really don't now. We have a model of illness, it's very much it's acute and time limited or it's fatal. And most people don't really have much sense of something in between. And there is very, very little understanding, I find in general about the concept of 'I can do that today, but not tomorrow', 'I could do this yesterday, but I can't do it today'. Or actually even more so, 'Yes, I can do that but the cost of doing so is so disproportionate that I need not to do it' … The notion that you will foot the bill later for stuff that you're doing now, and that you need to plan ahead for what happens as a result of the choices that you make today is just not the kind of planning that most people have to do or have ever had to do*" (Academic 12).

This approach to health impacts on academic practice and policy. For example, another of my interviewees described the process for reporting periods of ill health and how it impacted on her decision to work part-time: "*You had to go through a meeting with your supervisor where you had to go through 'Was this a recurring problem? Yes. Was there anything they could do? No. Was it going to happen again? Yes. Was there anything they could do? No'. And it's just a horrible tick box exercise and the form that people had to sign off. And it was just sort of like, do we have to do this every time. It's one of the reasons why I dropped down … I preferred losing two days of income a month to having to do those meetings twice a month*" (Academic 11).

The current focus on potential malingering is consistent with prominent media coverage of this issue. For example, Briant et al. (2013) document a 43% increase in disability-related media articles from 2004/5 to 2010/11. During this time media has become less sympathetic to disabled people and is increasingly likely to focus on entitlement to disability benefit and disability fraud. Illustrating the tone of these articles, the researchers demonstrate that news media are increasingly likely to use words such as "cheat" or "scrounger". This type of narrative has important consequences for the disclosure of a disability and access to disability services and accommodations. Indeed, Dorfman (2019) reports that nearly 60% of people with disabilities believe that others question their disability. This impacts on both those with visible and invisible conditions. It is often those who, whilst not disabled themselves, have a personal connection to disability (e.g. a loved one who is disabled) that are most suspicious and misguidedly attempt to "protect" facilities provided to support disabled people.

Olkin et al. (2019) describe the microaggressions experienced by women with disabilities, including people minimizing the impact of the disability on their life. Access to services is also problematic, with people that are not disabled often failing to appreciate the importance of accommodations, including viewing access to accessible parking spaces as a perk or bonus rather than essential support. As a consequence, disabled people may encounter a range of negative comments, stares, and questions when using services reserved for disabled people and the need to visibly demonstrate or prove their disability. As described by one woman, "Sometimes I get out of the car and I'm like, 'oh, who's around', like do I need to take out the wheelchair for show?" (p. 772). This issue impacts on both faculty members and students. For example, one student reported that the "Academic Dean informed me day before my exam that my exam provisions would be removed as I was 'doing too well'. I was horrified. 1) he didn't know the nature of my disability 2) this assumed that I doing really well is *beyond* my capabilities" (Osborne, 2019, p. 241).

These perceptions can lead to withdrawal and reluctance to engage with disabled facilities. As explained by one disabled person,

"I never reapplied for a parking plaque even though not having one has often caused me to avoid going to stores. If I can't get a close spot, sometimes I have to leave. I used to have one, but nearly every time I went out, I got verbally attacked, so it just became easier to adjust without one. I also avoid motorized carts for the same reasons. I have had people actually knock me down for the last cart; I've been attacked and berated all because I'm young and don't look disabled. I have congenital heart disease and Ehlers-Danlos syndrome along with incomplete paraplegia. Getting around is hard, getting a parking permit is harder, and actually using one is impossible" (Dorfman, 2019, p. 1082).

These issues apply to a range of facilities. As one of my interviewees explained: "*I went to the toilet and the only toilet there was a disabled one. And I went in it, and I just felt anxious and uncomfortable about having to leave it because, you know, I look fine. Luckily no one was there. But it just makes me feel bad. Like, I'm not justified in using it when I know I am. But I just feel bad about using it, I just feel guilty for my experiences sometimes*" (Academic 6).

Attempting to access disabled accommodations on public transport is especially difficult for those with invisible conditions and people with disabilities report being regularly challenged by members of the public. As recalled by one person, "I have gotten into fights with people around sitting in seats and … this one guy asked me like, 'what are you, pregnant? Do you need to be sitting here?' Or I've had older people like 'You need to get up because you know you can't sit there'" (Olkin et al., 2019, p. 772). As a consequence, people with disabilities often avoid using such facilities or only access them when carrying visible evidence of an impairment (e.g. mobility aids). For example, one member of faculty explained: "*I don't need to wear a mask, I'm in the exempt category at the moment. I always do if I go out because I wouldn't want to have to explain to somebody that I don't have to wear a mask. And if I get on a bus or train, not that I have done for months and months, I tend not to use the disabled seats and things like that. Because people would look at me and think, 'Well, she's not disabled', even though if I had to stand on the underground or stand on the bus even or go upstairs or something like that, some days would be quite an effort for me to do*" (Academic 5).

Some conditions (i.e. those where diagnosis depends on self-reports or test performance) appear to be especially subject to scrutiny, and the self-reported experiences (e.g. symptoms) of disabled people are often perceived to be less credible or legitimate than the reporting of a medical professional. Indeed, impairments may be dismissed by those without disabilities who state that they look "too healthy" or "too young" to be disabled (Olkin et al., 2019). Fluctuating and unpredictable conditions are especially susceptible to distrust and misunderstanding, and disabled people may be conscious that on one day they require support (e.g. accessible parking spaces) and on another they appear unaffected by the impairment. As described by one disabled woman, "I will be walking or something and then the next time that person sees me I'm going to be using my scooter and she will go, 'What happened?!' It's like you know like suddenly some horrible thing happened and I wasn't able to walk anymore. And then the next time they see me I will be walking and they would be 'well what's going on?' you know, it's like it's none of their business obviously" (Olkin et al., 2019, p. 773).

As a consequence, professional diagnosis is especially important for access to accommodations. As one of my interviewees recalled: "*It's bloody difficult to get a diagnosis and involved going private. But having it was such a huge improvement*" (Academic 3). These issues also impact on the experiences of disabled students who report both difficulty accessing accommodations without formal diagnosis and a fear that others perceive them to be lazy rather than impaired (Osborne, 2019). Comments from disabled students have included: "I have letters from multiple doctors stating that they believe that I do have a condition affecting sleep, but because I have no specific diagnosis, I don't get any support. I don't think University administrators realise that getting a diagnosis can take decades" (Osborne, 2019, p. 245), and "I'm not faking, I promise" (Osborne, 2019, p. 239). The reliance on professional diagnosis is, however, problematic, as a formal diagnosis or even recognition of a contested condition (e.g. lupus, chronic fatigue syndrome) can take many years. These issues are further exacerbated when medical professionals themselves do not believe people with disabilities (Olkin et al., 2019). It is essential, therefore, that access to accommodations is not dependent on formal diagnosis.

Summary

Perceptions of disability and specific conditions clearly impact on the lived experience of disabled people. Within academia, the attitudes held by students may have a substantial impact on the experience of disabled faculty. In this context, it is important to consider existing bias and the potential for disabled academics to positively impact on the attitudes and behaviour of others. Indeed, the presence of disabled academics appears to have a positive impact on both those who are and are not disabled.

Challenging perceptions: Disability simulation

Simulations of disability whereby people without disabilities "experience" disability represent one common intervention, intended to promote understanding and empathy. It is argued that simulations can provide personal insight into the lived experience of disability in an interesting and engaging format. These interventions may address both aspects of an individual impairment (e.g. simulating loss of vision) and structural barriers (e.g. requiring participants to navigate their way across campus whilst using a wheelchair). Disability simulations are most common for mobility or sensory impairments, for example, simulating wheelchair use or reduced sight or hearing. In contrast, simulations of other conditions, such as fatigue, can be more problematic, perhaps encouraging a narrow perception of what constitutes disability. Though these interventions are widely used, the use of simulations to educate people about disability has both advantages and disadvantages (Burgstahler & Doe, 2004; Herbert, 2000).

According to French (1992), disability simulations provide "a totally false impression of what it is like to be disabled" (p. 260). In part, this reflects the short-term nature of disability simulations, which provide limited insight into the nature of permanent disability or chronic health conditions. For example, they cannot convey the experience of fluctuating and unpredictable conditions. Leo and Goodwin (2016) explore the perceptions of wheelchair users on the use of disability simulations as a learning or training exercise. The disconnection between the reality of disability and the short-term simulated experience was highlighted as problematic. For example, one person reported:

> "I think the simulation is a great start, I don't think you could stop there. Like I see [at my school] where they get out of their chair and go 'Well, I'm done.' Great, like take the chair for like 24 hr and be in the chair really, go to the bar with the chair, see how tough it is to get a wheelchair cab back from the bar, and see how tough it is to get accessible transport, see how tough it is to get an accessible washroom at the bar, real stuff" (p. 166. Reprinted with permission from Leo & Goodwin, 2016. Simulating others' realities: Insiders reflect on disability simulations. *Adapted Physical Activity Quarterly*, 33(2), 156–175. https://doi.org/10.1123/APAQ.2015-0031).

Simulations can reduce the experience of disability to a caricature, that is intended to focus only on the deficits associated with a particular impairment. Indeed, there is typically little consideration of the strengths associated with disability or disability culture. As a consequence, participants may focus on initial feelings of distress, dependence, or vulnerability. For example, those participating in disability simulations have been reported to comment, "I would kill myself if I really had to stay in a wheelchair" and "This is awful!" (Grayson & Marini, 1996, p. 130). The distress experienced during simulation can encourage a fear of disability and subsequent avoidance of disabled people. As summarized by French (1992), "The focus on difficulties, problems and the disabled person's supposed inabilities and inadequacies is both inaccurate and depressing and gives rise to some very damaging stereotypes and misconceptions" (p. 260).

Those participating in a disability simulation on a short-term basis do not possess the coping strategies developed by disabled people. They may, therefore, internalize the belief that disabled people are less capable than non-disabled peers rather than appreciating the importance of accommodations or the strategies that disabled people develop to adapt to their condition. Unintended consequences could, therefore, include being less likely to employ disabled people who are perceived to be less able to complete required activities. It is, therefore, essential that simulations demonstrate the value of accommodations such as text to speech software. Arguably, the typical focus on making the simulation an enjoyable and engaging experience also reduces opportunities for more meaningful reflection and understanding. As stated by one wheelchair user, "The whole time they spent trying to get around with their friends and like it was a big game and it was fun, which is and it should be fun, but they're not really seeing what it really means to actually be in a chair" (Leo & Goodwin, 2016, p. 168. Reprinted with permission).

In part, difficulties with the implementation of disability simulations may reflect the lack of inclusion of disabled people with respect to the design and delivery of disability simulations. As stated by one wheelchair user:

> "You gotta involve the disability community. This is just harsh and you shouldn't take this personally ... but like, you shouldn't be teaching disability if you don't have the disability community involved. You just shouldn't. It's not right ... That's my criticism about simulations. If there's nobody with a disability involved in it, there's no value. Like, you're just wasting an opportunity for such great teaching. It's a wasted opportunity when you don't include the people with disabilities" (Leo & Goodwin, 2016, p. 165. Reprinted with permission).

Overall, there is little evidence that disability simulations are effective as an intervention designed to promote an understanding of disability in non-disabled groups (Flower et al., 2007). To an extent, this may reflect the fact that effective simulation of the disabled reality is unrealistic. As stated by Seropian (2003), "translating simulated experience into real experience is difficult if not impossible" (p. 1695). Simulations can, however, reveal important information about the beliefs held by non-disabled people towards those with disabilities.

In a series of experimental studies, Cohen et al. (2019) investigated the behaviour of people without disabilities when asked to simulate specific physical disabilities. In experimental conditions simulating a physical impairment, participants were asked to either wear filtered glasses (to represent visual impairment) or complete tasks whilst seated in a wheelchair. In the control condition, participants wore the filtered glasses (but there was no reference to disability) or were seated in a regular chair.

The participants simulating the impairment reported that they *felt* more disabled than those in the control condition, and they also completed the task more slowly. In one variation of the task, participants were asked to imagine that they were applying for a job, with the task and job interview completed whilst seated in a wheelchair or regular chair. Again, participants in the experimental condition reported feeling "more disabled" than those seated in a regular chair and performed more slowly. These findings demonstrate the extent to which people without disabilities expect disabled people to be less capable and effective than the non-disabled and that this is evident in both an artificial and more applied (i.e. employment) context.

7 Advice and guidance

There are a number of structural and operational issues that should be addressed in order to support faculty with disabilities. In this chapter, I provide a range of recommendations to address the systemic ableism that disadvantages disabled academics. Reflecting both the need to address structural discrimination within academia and the substantial labour that academics with disabilities already undertake to secure accommodations, recommendations focus on broad issues to be addressed by university management. These include recommendations based on the academic role (e.g. workload issues), accommodations (e.g. the process of disclosure), and support (e.g. disabled staff networks).

The academic role

The academic workload is problematic, with faculty often expected to work evenings and weekends to fulfil their roles and responsibilities (Houston et al., 2006). This practice contributes to a range of health and wellbeing issues amongst faculty (e.g. Melin et al., 2014; Pace et al., 2019; Sabagh et al., 2018) and negatively affects the retention of academic staff (Lindfelt et al., 2018). Highlighting the impact of traditional academic practice on self-care, health, and wellbeing, Beam and Clay-Buck (2018) comment that,

> "So much of 'working hard' is smoke and mirrors, created to fulfil artificial concepts of productivity rooted in outdated Puritanical ethics instead of what actually works well. When we internalize these ideas, we become fearful of our own needs and do not offer ourselves the same considerations we would anyone else" (p. 179).

Though these workload issues are challenging for all academics, they are especially likely to impede the wellbeing and career progression of disabled faculty. For example, one academic I interviewed commented: *"This idea that you know, a 40-hour work week should require roughly 60 hours of work. And if you can't fit it all in, then you are a bad employee and should do more of it in your own time. You know, people replying to emails all hours of the night, people getting up early to finish the work they didn't finish yesterday and I do it as well. They always estimate the work as taking less time than it does"* (Academic 11). Another stated: *"When I first took on the role, there was a bit of a buffer in terms of my own time as well that I could go, 'Okay, now's not a good day or even a good week'. And the work that I would do would be less but it would keep me healthier, and I wouldn't then progress to a sort of an overload situation that would then have a longer term impact on my health and ability to do that role. But now, there isn't that safety net, there isn't that fallback*" (Academic 1). Realistic workloads are necessary to promote academic wellbeing and reduce the incidence of long-term ill health.

In addition to their academic roles and responsibilities, disabled faculty often spend considerable time arranging workplace accommodations (Inckle, 2018). For example, disabled academics may spend time checking that their teaching rooms are accessible or learning to use specialist software. The time required to arrange accommodations and complete particular tasks (e.g. marking when using specialist software) is not typically taken into consideration when calculating academic workloads or allocating roles and responsibilities. As summarized by one interviewee: "*A student with an individual learning plan will get an extended deadline. So in some cases, automatic extensions for submission of the work, and will get additional time allowance for completion of that work. But a member of staff who has the same or similar condition, won't get additional time for marking it*" (Academic 1). It is essential that the additional work undertaken by disabled scholars is considered and addressed in workload models. If this does not occur, disabled faculty are systematically disadvantaged compared to their non-disabled colleagues.

Standard criteria for the evaluation of academic performance typically focuses on a range of highly specific activities. Indeed, academia often fails to acknowledge alternative forms of education practice. This approach both limits the opportunity for educational innovation and disadvantages those with specific impairments. As described by one of my interviewees: "*A lot of the major scientific breakthroughs are dyslexic because they weren't forced into conformity. And I just feel that academia forces you to conform to what is a read-write environment and anything that talks about neurodiversity is fine until then we legitimize it through publications, and its publication in these journals. Really? Can't we move away from that? Can't we do something different? And I think for me, it's the problem of what is accepted and what is perceived as legitimate, you know, for academia. And it's still so read-write. And it's still very, very controlled by people who think that way*" (Academic 2). Disabled faculty should be supported by providing greater flexibility in their role. For example, Beam and Clay-Buck (2018) describe their own teaching practice, referred to as "low-spoon" teaching. This approach both accommodates their own needs (e.g. reducing energy expenditure) and benefits the student cohort (e.g. students demonstrated greater agency and a more collaborative approach with faculty).

Promotion

Programmes created to support disabled employees often focus on recruitment rather than promotion. It is, however, important to address issues relating to career advancement and ensure that disabled faculty are supported to secure leadership positions. In this context, it is important to note that disabled employees are often infantilized (Nario-Redmond et al., 2019) and denied opportunities to develop or excel. It is essential that disabled faculty are offered the same opportunities to engage in challenging and demanding activities that contribute to career advancement and progression as their non-disabled colleagues. It is also important to acknowledge that disabled people may develop a number of transferable skills that enhance their leadership role. As explained by one academic, "All my life I have had to solve problems. I'm a disabled person navigating a world designed by non-disabled people. I think laterally and encourage other people to do the same. My approach to leadership is inevitably informed by my approach to life" (Martin, 2017, p. 14). Of course, whilst recognizing and developing the skills of disabled faculty, it is also important to create academic roles and opportunities for those with disabilities (Mellifont et al., 2019).

Academic promotion typically involves a lengthy application and review process during which the applicant must demonstrate that they are already working at the desired level (i.e. above and beyond their current role). To demonstrate this level of performance, academics may take on a range of additional roles and responsibilities (e.g. external examiner, journal editor) that exceed their allocated workload. Indeed, those adopting long working hours are more likely to secure academic promotion (Beasley et al., 2006). Of course, the expectation that academics work excessive hours (including evenings and weekends) discriminates against those unable to do so, such as those with caring responsibilities or energy-limiting conditions. As summarized by one interviewee: *"I've actually made the decision, and it's totally wrong. But I've made the decision that, for instance, I'm not even considering going for any promotions. Because the remit for getting a promotion at our university, is that you have to be seen to go above and beyond your usual role ... I'm like, 'Well tell me how I can meet the criteria for promotion without actually doing additional work above my current role'. And nobody's got any answers"* (Academic 1). It is essential that promotion is achievable for those unable to work excessive hours and the additional difficulties experienced by disabled faculty (e.g. the accessibility of academic conferences) are taken into consideration.

Part-time roles and precarious contracts

For faculty unable to engage in full-time work, part-time contracts may be more appropriate. These may, however, restrict career progression. As one part-time faculty member explained: *"Okay, I'm only ever going to be able to work part-time. Well, that's Professor right off the list. You know that because all of the methods of career building are based on this idea you'll be working, you know, six if not seven days a week. You know, the way we think about productivity, the way we look at people's CVs and judge their output is based on this idea that they will be working a full-time week that you do just have to accept, okay, even if I work to my limit, I'm only going to be able to get through 60% of the career and that is distressing and annoying, and makes me very frustrated"* (Academic 11). It is essential that part-time positions are both available and supported and that part-time academics have the same opportunities for promotion as their full-time colleagues. It is important to recognize here that whilst failure to acknowledge the achievements of part-time employees clearly impacts on individual academics, it also negatively impacts on the institution by excluding experienced and capable faculty from senior leadership roles. It is, therefore, in the best interests of the institution to address these issues.

Academia is increasingly characterized by precarious (fixed-term and casual) contracts. The negative impact of precarious employment on the careers and personal life of employees has been well documented (Bozzon et al., 2017). For disabled academics, precarious contracts present additional challenges. For example, increased competition for academic positions and the need to frequently apply for teaching or research contracts heighten reputational concerns. Academics may avoid disclosing a disability or requesting accommodations in order to avoid the stigma and discrimination associated with disability. Indeed, the impact of disability on hiring decisions is well documented (Ameri et al., 2018). As a consequence, faculty who feel unable to disclose an impairment cannot obtain the support that they require. For those who are prepared to disclose, frequently changing roles, institutions, or regions involves more frequent disclosure and requests for accommodations, requiring substantial time and emotional labour. Precarious contracts can also disrupt access to health care, medical insurance, and self-care routines. Academia must address the widespread use of precarious contracts and the negative impact of these on disabled faculty.

Research publication, funding, and assessment

Publication

Publication is central to the Neoliberal assessment of academic performance and promotion criteria (Dobele & Rundle-Theile, 2015), though the focus on journal outputs arguably leaves little time for other important activities such as creativity and reflection (Fischer et al., 2012). The emphasis placed on publication in peer-reviewed journals may be especially problematic for some faculty members. For example, publication in traditional academic journals may be more challenging for academics who are Deaf, reflecting the different grammatical structures of written and sign languages. In addition, there may be fewer opportunities for co-authorship on collaborative research projects and the support and mentoring programmes that are typically provided to academics may be less accessible to Deaf faculty. The advantages gained by Deaf doctoral students with access to a mentor who is familiar with sign language have been documented, though opportunities for such mentoring programmes are limited and require expansion (Braun et al., 2017).

Marchut et al. (2021) describe the development of an intensive five-day writing retreat for Deaf academics. All instruction was provided in American Sign Language (ASL) and DeafSpace recommendations (Edwards & Harold, 2014) were adopted (e.g. ensuring that the lighting and furniture allow clear communication between participants). The programme both highlighted the issues experienced by Deaf faculty and provided structured support. As described by one mentor,

> "Many of our participants have a fear of judgment that comes with writing ... You can be told you are 'no good' so many times before it becomes part of one's reality. I think the blocks Deaf writers have are largely psychological. They are not actual blocks as a matter of ability" (Marchut et al., 2021, p. 186).

It is important to emphasize that difficulties surrounding journal publication are not limited to Deaf faculty. For example, publication may also be more difficult for dyslexic academics. As described by one of my interviewees: "*If I'm told, you know, you will be expected to produce two journal articles a year, that is going to disable me. If they say you're supposed to just disseminate your work and the value of my dissemination is quantified to let you know, you'll do X amount of webinars on that, then that won't disable me*" (Academic 2). These issues must be recognized, with greater support available and a more flexible approach to research dissemination adopted.

Funding

Researchers able to secure grant funding are more likely to achieve promotion (Bloch et al., 2014). Considerable prestige is also attached to research funding. For example, one academic described the extent to which a grant had "helped strengthen my position as a researcher, making it easier to secure collaboration partners for research projects and leading to invitations to hold lectures and participate in meetings based on one's own work. So, the grant has meant a great deal and helped open a lot of doors" (Bloch et al., 2014, p. 92). There is, however, substantial bias in the review of grant applications and allocation of grant funding (Morgan et al., 2018). It is important to address such bias both with respect to the allocation of research funding and the prestige that is attached to grant funding vs. other activities.

There are a number of barriers experienced by disabled faculty applying for research funding. For example, preparing the grant application may be more difficult for some researchers (see previous section for barriers experienced by Deaf and dyslexic faculty). In addition, disabled academics may be required to request specific resources that makes the grant application more costly and therefore less competitive compared with the applications submitted by their non-disabled colleagues. For example, additional support may be required to facilitate attendance at meetings or conferences (interpreters, carers, etc.) or the range of suitable options (e.g. accessible hotel accommodation and transport) may be more limited. It is important that funders provide the required support to disabled faculty but that they do so in a way that does not penalize disabled applicants. In particular, grants that include disability-related costs should not be perceived as less competitive than applications that do not require workplace accommodations.

Some academics may receive funding to complete their postgraduate (e.g. PhD) studies. Although students are required to enrol on a full-time or part-time basis, some disabled students may be unable to work on a full-time basis but unable to cope financially on a part-time (0.5) contract. Additional options (e.g. 0.7 contracts), therefore, would likely be beneficial. Similarly, postgraduate funders should acknowledge that some students may need to suspend their studies more frequently than others and require support for activities typically completed by the student themselves (e.g. interview transcription). It is also important to recognize that part-time contracts are typically intended for students engaged in additional paid employment (e.g. teaching). Disabled students may not be able to engage in additional work, placing them at a considerable disadvantage, both with regards to their financial security and the work experience obtained. These issues should be acknowledged when monitoring student progress and treated sympathetically by potential employers.

One of my interviewees spoke as follows: "*There is zero credit for what working or studying with these kinds of restrictions actually involves, in the way there is for other people whose time for study is limited for other reasons. Like if you're holding down a full-time job, and you're doing a full-time PhD, you get huge amounts of kudos for that. Everybody sort of goes, 'Wow, impressive, you are a driven and committed individual, good on you. And by the way, you're also simultaneously getting bonus employment experience that will make you more likely to get a job' ... I will never, ever, ever get any credit for the fact that I'm going to finish a PhD in under four years on 50% hours. Never. I can't even say it because saying that would make me less credible. The commitment and drive it takes for me to do this makes me less credible as an employee, because I can't put in as many hours. If I were doing this part-time, I would be finishing before my point of minimum candidature. And I would get a lot of credit for that. But because I'm doing it part time, all you see when you look at my CV is well it took four years to do it. Only done this many conferences, only got two papers in press, you know. If I were working full time, the amount that I could do would set me way above most of my peers. And that ability is not reflected on paper, or anywhere that anybody will ever see it. And it's not fair. I'm so much better than most of most of my able-bodied peers, and you can't see it and nobody will ever give me any credit for it. You don't benefit from it. It's just enraging, the invisibility of not just the disability but the work that goes into performing is never contextualized. And one can't contextualize it, because to do so makes you less credible*" (Academic 12).

Assessment and metrics

The inadequacy of current metric-based performance assessments has been acknowledged. In particular, these have been criticized for the narrow indicators of "success" considered by such metrics and the systemic bias that exists. Davies et al. (2021) conclude: "These metrics are flawed and biased against already marginalized groups and fail to accurately capture the breadth of individuals' meaningful scientific impacts. We advocate shifting this outdated value system to advance science through principles of justice, equity, diversity and

Advice and guidance 89

inclusion" (p. 1). These same authors propose more inclusive definitions of success and impact that value a range of academic activities, including science communication, community engagement, and collaboration. Further, they contrast the current academic culture that restricts equality and diversity and reduces innovation with a more collaborative and inclusive model that promotes academic wellbeing.

Accommodation and inclusive design

Employers often adopt the attitude that "No one in my team is disabled so I don't need to think about accessibility. I will make adjustments later if I need to." As summarized by one interviewee: *"There's often a thing of 'Well, we'll plan for it if it comes up.' But if you leave that planning to 'if it comes up' it's too late"* (Academic 11). The failure to consider disability can create a hostile environment for people with disabilities. As described by one faculty member I interviewed: *"I'm in a relatively new building … the doors to get into the open plan area are full wall height … they are really, really heavy … So anyone who has less than normal strength and use of their arms, and hands and legs and everything, couldn't even go to the toilet without asking someone. The toilets are the other side of those doors. So you couldn't even get in. There are disabled toilets with a shower, but you couldn't get to them without asking someone to help you get to them. There's no automatic doors in the building except the one to get actually into the reception area. That's it"* (Academic 5). It is, therefore, essential for institutions to raise the profile of disability in order to ensure that the academic environment is accessible to those with disabilities.

As discussed in Chapter 4, faculty may be reluctant to disclose an impairment. For example, they may decide to assess the attitudes of their colleagues or line manager before making themselves vulnerable to workplace discrimination. As a consequence, it is unlikely that employers would be aware of all disabled employees (or, of course, be able to predict future impairments). In addition, many employees may experience short-term impairment (e.g. depleted energy or concentration) as a consequence of short-term illness or the side effects of medication. Adopting an inclusive and accessible approach that extends beyond those disabled employees known to employers is, therefore, most appropriate and likely to support a wide range of faculty members. Universal Design represents a proactive and inclusive approach. In essence, Universal Design anticipates the presence of people with disabilities and embeds accessibility in the planning process, reducing the need for individual retrospective accommodations (Dolmage, 2015).

Universal Design for Learning is more frequently discussed in relation to disabled students than disabled faculty (e.g. Gradel & Edson, 2009). The concerns of academics implementing Universal Design to support the student experience are also commonly discussed (e.g. LaRocco & Wilken, 2013; Westine et al., 2019). Indeed, universities appear to be less equipped (or willing) to support disabled faculty compared to their support for disabled students

(Smith & Andrews, 2015). In part, this may reflect a reluctance to accept that disabled people can become academics. As summarized by one of my interviewees: *"… that crosses over with other learning difficulties, like dyslexia, which universities, culturally speaking, assume is a problem that 18-year-old students have, and then, then just miraculously stop being dyslexic. You know, maybe they'll do a Master's, but like, the concept that there will be academics with additional learning needs, it's just kind of [uses hands and facial expression to indicate mind blown], it's mind-blowing stuff for a lot of people. Which is bananas to me, because I think that a lot of the traits that make me good at what I do come from my learning disability. Actually I'm creative and I have interesting ideas because of the way ADHD means that I think, I don't regret that at all"* (Academic 12).

There may also be uncertainty with regards to the type of accommodations available. As one interviewee commented: *"Anything that's outside of that mainstream of Deaf, Blind, wheelchair, you know, the ones they put on the symbols so you know someone's disabled. Anything that's fluctuating, anything that is a little odd, it can be very hard to get people to understand. And then once they understand, to put in an appropriate level of assistance. Like initially in my current job, I was banned from working evenings and weekends, even though I had flexi time, because they were worried about what if I fell asleep and there was a fire and it's like, 'I wake up, I'm not unconscious, it's sleep. Like it doesn't matter how foggy headed I am I can get out of a burning building'"* (Academic 11). Making the range of potential accommodations clear (e.g. using fictional examples to illustrate appropriate accommodations and how to access these) would be beneficial. There may also be inconsistency in the way in which accommodations are approved. For example, some people report using their "clout" to access accommodations (Stone et al., 2013) and it is important to ensure that support is available to all staff regardless of role or status.

Disabled employees report difficulties when accommodations are perceived to be a "favour" or dependent on the actions of a single line manager. This approach requires further negotiation if a new line manager is appointed or a restructure takes place. This system is also open to abuse, with decisions potentially influenced by the personal attitudes of line managers in relation to individual employees or specific impairments (Balser, 2007). As summarized by one faculty member: *"You can't make access a personal favour. Because as soon as it's a personal favour, and it's not enshrined in sort of the institutional codes or in law as it were, that means that this person's ability to access their workplace is contingent on the goodwill of other members of staff and their peers. The reason I had no redress is because it was a personal favour, I didn't have an actual right to be in this space, which is totally unacceptable. You can't make that sort of thing contingent on goodwill. And as long as it's done as a personal favour as sort of like, 'Oh, we'll just tweak it for you', as soon as that manager changes, or somebody takes exception, as soon as the situation changes, you lose all of your rights to even remotely equal treatment. And that is not what equality looks like, at all. That just means that you can't possibly ever annoy anybody ever. Because your presence is a favour"* (Academic 12). Universities should review procedure to ensure that appropriate accommodations (e.g. those recommended by Occupational Health) cannot be denied by individual line managers.

Securing accommodations, diagnosis, and disclosure

Employers must recognize not only that they have a legal obligation to provide appropriate workplace accommodations but the positive impact of doing so. For example, accommodations enable employees to be more productive and enhance employee recruitment and retention (Hartnett et al., 2011; Solovieva et al., 2011). It is important, therefore, to address barriers that limit access to these accommodations. In particular, employees are often expected to provide "proof" of their impairment in order to access workplace accommodations (Gold et al., 2012). People with disabilities may, however, experience a considerable delay between the onset of symptoms and professional diagnosis (e.g. Choy et al., 2010; Hadfield et al., 1996). As a consequence, many disabled faculty may not have the required medical evidence to secure workplace accommodations. Accommodations should not be dependent on medical diagnosis. Indeed, reliance on medical diagnosis may undermine the importance of the individual's lived experience (Olsen et al., 2020).

As described by one of my interviewees: *"I've got no diagnosis for the fatigue stuff like other than where it comes under the fibromyalgia umbrella. But I mean, why would they bother to diagnose it? They've got no treatments for it, there's nothing useful down that diagnosis path, so they don't bother going down it. Which is useful in that you don't go to a bunch of appointments that are fundamentally useless but also frustrating from the point of view that you have fewer labels. And labels are very helpful in getting people to recognize what it is rather than the cluster of symptoms whereas the cluster of symptoms should be enough, right? You shouldn't need a name for it. If it's been happening to you for a year and they can't do anything about it, you shouldn't need a label to convince your work that this is something they have to adapt for. Particularly because the labels are [long pause] a bit arbitrary in a lot of places. Like do I have fatigue because I have a fatigue condition or do I have fatigue because my pain meds increase my slightly natural tendency toward fatigue. It doesn't really matter, right. The problem is the same either way. The thing we have to deal with is the fatigue"* (Academic 11).

In addition, there appears to be a "hierarchy" of conditions, with some impairments perceived to be more acceptable, legitimate, or deserving of support (Freeze et al., 1999). Some conditions (e.g. Lyme disease, chronic fatigue syndrome) are especially contested and may be dismissed by both the medical profession and wider society (Hinds & Sutcliffe, 2019). For example, chronic fatigue syndrome has been historically labelled as 'yuppie flu' in the popular press (de Wolfe, 2009). As a consequence, some individuals may experience considerable delay receiving diagnosis and medical care or be cautious when revealing the name of their condition. It is essential, therefore, that academics are supported to receive workplace accommodations during the pre-diagnosis phase. Similarly, people who have a negative experience with the medical profession may cease engagement with the medical community or avoid further assessment. Workplace accommodations that are reliant on diagnosis (or other assessments such as the Blue Badge scheme) are likely to exclude a substantial number of disabled employees; access to support should not be reliant on these. For example, priority parking may benefit those with energy-limiting conditions regardless of the final diagnosis or engagement with the Blue Badge scheme.

To secure workplace accommodations (or when providing basic demographic information), academics are typically required to self-identify as disabled. Of course, the term "disability" is not value free and many people who meet the legal criteria for disability may not identify as disabled (Watson, 2002). For example, individuals may not consider their condition to be a disability. Alternatively, people may avoid the term disabled because of the stigma associated with disability or because they do not consider themselves to be "disabled enough". As one interviewee commented: "*I haven't actually registered with disability. I've mentioned it, but when it says on a form, are you disabled or not? I was like, well, not at the moment, sort of. I don't know how to answer that. I definitely have been in the past where it would have majorly impacted me. But now it's sort of okay*" (Academic 7).

Standard reporting procedures are, therefore, problematic if academics are required to "declare a disability" in order to access support. This practice requires those who do not identify as disabled to either accept an identity that does not represent their experience or not access appropriate accommodations. Institutions should consider the language used when gathering demographic information and when facilitating access to workplace accommodations. Processes must be appropriate for employees with a range of conditions and those who do not personally identify as disabled. For example, rather than "Are you disabled?" or "Do you consider yourself to have a disability?", questions such as "Do you have additional support needs?" or "Are there adjustments that would support you?" may be more appropriate. As described by one interviewee: "*It's a hard line to know when to disclose that information I think because I was never asked. The only option is 'Do you have a disability?' or 'Do you have any mental health conditions?' Well, no, I don't. But are you going to give me another option? Like, 'Do you feel like you need additional support?'*" (Academic 6). Of course, the language used to obtain disability-related information also has important ramifications beyond the individual disclosing. For example, universities with relatively few employees disclosing a disability may be unwilling to invest in disabled staff networks.

Funding accommodations

Employers are often concerned that workplace accommodations will be financially costly, even though most accommodations do not require funding (Smith & Andrews, 2015). Where financial investment is required, it is important that accommodations are centrally funded by the university rather than financed by a specific academic department. This reduces the possibility that line managers will refuse an accommodation because of limited departmental funds. Centralizing funding also reduces the likelihood that non-disabled colleagues who believe that accommodations negatively impact funds available for other activities (e.g. conference attendance or training) will display resentment (Woodcock et al., 2007).

It is important to recognize that people with disabilities often incur substantial personal costs, for example assistive devices, medication, and rehabilitation (Mitra et al., 2017). It is especially important, therefore, that academics with disabilities are not expected to personally fund workplace accommodations. Furthermore, academics with disabilities often spend a great deal of time securing accommodations and necessary support (Inckle, 2018). As described by one academic, "… I spent about three days a week – three full-time days a week – arranging my own travel, booking it all, researching it, filling my university claims – because everything has to be claimed through the university first – and then the Access to Work claim. Each one is a three-stage process …" (Merchant et al., 2020, p. 281). Universities should review current systems to ensure that disabled academics are not required to fund their own accommodations and that they are compensated for time arranging these.

Specific impairments and disciplines

Specific impairments may present particular challenges. For example, Smith and Andrews (2015) provide suggestions for those working with hearing-impaired academics. These suggestions include seating individuals in a circle that provides open lines of sight between contributors and ensuring that only one person speaks at a time. Brown (2021) provides personal accounts of a range of impairments together with recommendations for practice focused on each condition. Universities should familiarize themselves with good practice associated with specific impairments. It is important to understand, however, that people with the same condition may require different workplace accommodations. The necessary accommodations will be influenced by issues including (but not limited to) the degree of impairment, existence of co-morbid conditions, the academic role and responsibilities, and personal circumstance. Effective accommodations can only be provided following discussion with the disabled academic themselves. It is also important to recognize that it may be difficult for those with disabilities to anticipate the accommodations or equipment that will be most beneficial and ongoing support should be provided.

As summarized by one member of faculty: *"The way work react to the request for equipment is that you've got to get it right first time. If you need a specialist chair, don't come back in two months saying, 'This one doesn't work for me, can I try a different one?' You need to know, somehow magically, what the right chair is that's going to fit the condition, what the mouse is that's going to solve your hands. They'll ask you for the accommodations you need. And you need to be right the first time because if you try and change them later, and they've already spent money on them, they will be so grumpy*" (Academic 11). Therefore, faculty must be supported to secure new accommodations if the original support provided is not sufficient. Of course, whilst universities are likely to focus their attention on the accommodations provided to academics based at their own institution, external visitors may also have additional requirements. Normalizing the provision of disability-specific information creates a more inclusive environment and should be encouraged. For example, when providing external visitors with a map of the university campus, information detailing accessible routes should be included.

It is important to recognize that specific disciplines or activities may present particular challenges for disabled academics (e.g. fieldwork). Discussing the need to undergo a National Health Service (NHS) medical examination to demonstrate their fitness to complete a research project, one researcher explained: "The biggest problem for me has been the way that the individualized vetting and surveillance procedures have re-awakened my own deep-seated fears around being judged solely on the basis of my impairment" (Tregaskis & Goodley, 2005, p. 371). Furthermore: "My previous largely negative experiences with the medical profession made me suspect they would be looking for any reason they could that was connected to my impairment to deny me permission to do the research" (Tregaskis & Goodley, 2005, p. 371). Disabled academics must be supported to navigate these issues. Universities should also acknowledge the anxiety associated with some activities or systems.

Employers must be mindful that some disciplines or courses (e.g. psychology, medicine, nursing, social work, law) are likely to include specific issues of representation. The way in which impairments, disability, and disabled people are discussed may have a considerable impact on the way in which academics and students view a condition and act towards those with that impairment. For disabled academics and students, the content of these sessions (and the accompanying materials or reading) provide an indication of how the discipline, institution, and potentially their peers feel about disability or specific impairments, and how they may react to disclosure. That is not to say that an open discussion cannot be held about specific impairments or disability (which may be beneficial to challenge existing bias or misconceptions) but this should be held in a respectful, informed, and progressive manner. For example, care should be taken to address common stereotypes that demonize or infantilize disability.

Many academic disciplines benefit from the involvement of experts by experience (e.g. service users). For example, Comensus (Community Engagement and Service User Support) at the University of Central Lancashire (UK) embeds the service user and carer voice across numerous departments (https://www.uclan.ac.uk/values-and-initiatives/comensus). These experts by experience can provide a more nuanced account of a disability than the list of symptoms typically prioritized in textbook accounts. Experts by experience also highlight the lived experience of specific impairments, including the importance of the diagnosis, consultation, and treatment process. Universities should provide experts by experience with the same status as academic experts by ensuring that their insight informs each stage of provision (e.g. curriculum design and course review). Similarly, when the institution hosts events such as an academic conference, the attendance of experts by experience strengthens this provision.

The contribution of disabled people to academic practice and policy should not be limited to teaching or research related to specific impairments or disability. For example, a recent review of higher education policy (Khan, 2021) revealed that although disabled academics and students are more likely to experience domestic abuse than their non-disabled peers, relatively few universities in the UK have a specific domestic abuse policy and even fewer recognize the additional needs required by those with disabilities. It is essential that disabled people are considered and represented in all aspects of higher education in order that their needs are fully met in a range of contexts.

Academic conferences and events

Attendance and presentation at academic conferences provide a range of benefits. For example, academics can disseminate their research, engage in scientific debate, and learn about important opportunities such as vacant committee positions. As a consequence, conferences have been described as "a vital part of academic life" (Sousa & Clark, 2017, p. 1). Academic conferences are not, however, equally accessible for all faculty. For example, women attend fewer conferences than their male colleagues and are more likely to attend local than international conferences (Timperley et al., 2020).

Female delegates are also more likely to report negative conference experiences such as discrimination or harassment. Commenting on academic conference attendance, one academic stated: "On several occasions, I have experienced mostly male colleagues treat the Annual Meeting (and other PS conferences) like their personal playground and the women who attend it – including graduate students – as their weekend dating pool". Another commented: "being a young woman scholar at APSA is often exhausting. The harassment is nearly constant, from men who stare at your chest rather than your eyes while you're speaking to explicit propositioning after a few drinks at a reception" (Sapiro & Campbell, 2018, p. 202).

Disabled academics also report negative conference experiences. For example, one of my interviewees stated: *"Conferences are phenomenally exhausting. I think I could be quite happy never going to a conference again"* (Academic 3). Another explained: *"I just find it too long a day ... Sometimes they can start at eight o'clock, sometimes with meetings, pre meeting meetings, you know. Some committee meetings and things like that. Or they'll have meetings during lunch as well. So you know, you don't actually stop for lunch. And even, well I'm sure you've been to meetings, even when you have a tea break, you're not actually having a break. It's you're stood up and you have to chat to other people and talk about science and you know, things like that so it's not actually a break ... So you start at maybe eight o'clock, and you're still going at half ten, 11 o'clock*" (Academic 5).

Demonstrating the extent to which conference accessibility is problematic, access issues are also apparent at disability-focused conferences (Callus, 2017). Indeed, Hodge (2014) reports that some delegates are "encouraged to self-exclude; their life at conference is made uncomfortable through demonstrations by other delegates and conference 'officials' of frustration, annoyance, irritation and other similar acts of veiled aggression" (p. 656). Therefore, it is important that conference organizers expect and anticipate that disabled academics will attend and present at conferences rather than seek to make only ad-hoc accommodations if individual delegates raise access issues. This is consistent with the Universal Design approach discussed earlier in this chapter. It is also important to bear in mind that whilst guidance for conference inclusivity often focuses on the conference venue, conference organizers must attend to the accessibility of the overall conference experience. For example, calls for abstracts and conference registration should be available in accessible formats.

Conference accommodation and accessibility

National and international conferences are often hosted by a different institution each year, requiring each new committee to locate a venue for the conference and suitable hotel accommodation. When choosing a venue, conference organizers are likely to consider a range of factors, including the financial cost and aesthetic or historic appeal of the building. It is important that conference venues are accessible, including the time taken to move between parallel sessions. As one interviewee commented: "*The whole thing was very much in that technically accessible space, in that technically I could get to every room, but it involved going out and up a lift and down and out. And that involves having someone to come and open the door because they kept wedging half the door shut for environmental reasons in the college*" (Academic 11). The availability of accessible transport and hotel accommodation is also important. For example, accessible hotel rooms must be both affordable and convenient to travel to the conference venue. Often, accessible rooms are available only at expensive hotels creating an additional barrier for disabled scholars.

Conference delegates may ask for specific accommodations. However, others may not feel comfortable disclosing this information. Indeed, though managers or colleagues from a delegate's own institution may not be in attendance, by their nature conferences address a specific subject discipline and delegates may be reluctant to disclose an impairment to research collaborators, those likely to review publications or grant proposals, and potential employers. It is important, therefore, to anticipate the presence of disabled faculty and create an accessible and inclusive environment. Where accommodations or additional support are requested, delegates should not be expected to justify this (e.g. with medical details or diagnosis). Examples of measures that can be taken to improve conference accessibility include ensuring that all speakers (including those that introduce presentations or make conference announcements) use microphones. Often, speakers in small venues simply state, "I assume everyone can hear me without the microphone" or ask, "Does anyone need me to use the microphone?". Disabled delegates should not feel pressurized to publicly declare a hearing impairment, with the emphasis on inclusive design that is accessible for all delegates.

Where it is not possible to make adjustments, alternative solutions should be sought. For example, if the height of the lectern cannot be adjusted for wheelchair users, clickers may allow presenters to move between slides without needing to return to the lectern. A range of technologies are available to support conference accessibility. For example, live captions may be used. When using technologies (e.g. live captioning and live streaming) it is important to ensure that the technologies selected are compatible. These captions should also be available to those who are unable to attend on the day or viewing in a breakout room. A large number of conference organizers or volunteers are, of course, required to monitor different aspects of the conference, including reliability of the live captioning.

Increasingly, conferences have recognized the importance of invisible or non-visible disabilities. For example, some conferences provide quiet rooms that are of benefit for a range of delegates, including those experiencing sensory overload or with energy-limiting conditions. These typically feature low lighting and provide a comfortable place to rest (e.g. with blankets and cushions included). Additional measures to support conference activities include ensuring that chairs are available during poster presentations and displaying posters throughout the conference (rather than a narrow time slot), allowing delegates to view these when they are most comfortable (e.g. when the area is quieter and less crowded). It is important to acknowledge that delegates may have a range of requirements or co-morbid conditions that should be accommodated. For example, quiet rooms created to support those with energy-limiting or sensory issues should also be wheelchair accessible.

It may of course be difficult for conference organizers to anticipate all issues. For example, conference organizers may provide interpreters for formal presentations but fail to provide interpreters who can facilitate communication during informal networking sessions. The lack of interpreters during networking sessions effectively excludes Deaf conference attendees from opportunities to discuss their work, learn about new opportunities, or form research collaborations. Involving disabled academics in conference organization is important. For example, Deaf academics are likely to anticipate such issues together with the importance of providing appropriate rest breaks for those interpreters. It is also important that conference spaces are regularly reviewed to ensure that accessibility has not been compromised. For example, delegates may move chairs or furniture during a session, rendering the space inaccessible to wheelchair users.

Academic conferences typically provide light refreshments and lunches. Buffet lunches that require delegates to carry food and drink can be problematic for disabled academics (e.g. those carrying mobility aids or with coordination difficulties). Similarly, delegates are often expected to stand when eating buffet lunches, which is difficult for some attendees (e.g. those with energy-limiting conditions) and less inclusive for wheelchair users (De Picker, 2020). Therefore, a seated lunch with individuals pre-selecting their food may be more appropriate. For example, Brown et al. (2018) describe the organization of a conference in which food and drink options were delivered to tables. Colour-coded stickers on delegate badges may be one relatively straightforward approach to assign the correct food options. Where food cannot be pre-selected, it should be clearly labelled to support those with allergies and specific dietary requirements. Where specific requests are made, it is important that these are treated seriously, and delegates are not questioned about their reasons for avoiding specific food types. Caterers may also provide alcohol (e.g. at welcome drinks receptions or during a poster presentation evening) which can be difficult for those with substance use issues. It is important to provide a range of non-alcoholic alternatives and ensure that delegates do not feel othered when avoiding alcohol or pressurized to justify their abstinence.

The issues outlined in this section are not an exhaustive list. For example, to ensure that a conference is fully inclusive, the principles of Universal Design should also be applied to related social events (e.g. conference dinners and organized tours of the host city). For additional guidance on accessible conferences, see Brown and colleagues' (2018) description of creating an accessible and inclusive event and De Picker's (2020) account of conference attendance as a disabled scholar. Of course, whilst this section focuses on disability in relation to in-person conference attendance, the COVID-19 pandemic has highlighted the utility of online conferences and their potential to improve accessibility (Rich et al., 2020). It is important, however, that where both online and offline attendance is supported, this does not result in a "two-tier" system whereby online and offline delegates receive access to formal presentations but only those attending in-person have access to networking opportunities, etc.

Mentoring, support, and disabled staff networks

Mentoring programmes have been successfully used to support academic progression. For example, in one mentoring programme developed to support female academics, mentees obtained higher grant income, achieved higher levels of promotion, and were more likely to remain at the university (Gardiner et al., 2007). As described in Chapter 6, mentors can also provide valuable support to disabled academics. It is important that universities provide such programmes and these should not be restricted to those in the early stages of their career. Networking programmes should also be provided to support the career progression of disabled faculty. Institutional mentoring and networking programmes are especially important for disabled academics, as traditional networking opportunities (e.g. conferences) are less accessible to disabled faculty (De Picker, 2020; Williams & Mavin, 2015).

For academics who become disabled, this change in circumstance can be distressing. Counselling can provide academics with the required support. As described by one of my interviewees: "*I ended up about two years ago taking part in some counselling, because I just found like, my life had really changed since the Lyme disease and I don't think I'd really given myself time to process that I went straight from being in hospital when I was first diagnosed, to straight back to work. And had never really stopped to kind of say, you know what, it's okay to be sad about this. And, you know, your life has changed, it's okay to admit that and process that*" (Academic 8). Counselling should be available to all academic staff. This support should not incur a cost and should be accessible without direct requests to line managers. Disabled staff networks can also provide support to disabled academics. This may include informal support, guidance on disability-relevant university systems, and collective advocacy for disabled employees. The National Association of Disabled Staff Networks (NADSN, https://www.nadsn-uk.org/) can provide support, guidance, and resources for existing networks or for those wishing to create a new Disabled Staff Network.

Where disabled staff networks are available, activities often focus on practical issues and disabled advocacy (e.g. addressing the accessibility of the university campus), with relatively little consideration of disability culture. Indeed, although universities often provide centres to recognize and celebrate specific cultural groups (e.g. international students), few institutions create centres that are focused on disability culture, preferring to focus on impairment and accommodations to address this (e.g. interpreters or note-takers). Chiang (2020) describes the introduction of a Disability Cultural Center at the University of North Carolina Asheville. Such centres support the development of a disabled community, allowing individuals to socialize, support each other, and campaign for disability rights. Universities should seek to raise the profile of disability culture and integrate this within provision for disabled academics and students.

Education and training

Diversity training specific to disability is required (Jones, 1997). This training should challenge common stereotypes related to disability (e.g. that disabled people are dependent or dangerous). Disability-related training initiatives often adopt a deficit approach, focusing on negative aspects of the impairment, such as poor coordination or difficulty maintaining concentration. Whilst it is important to recognize issues that may require accommodation, the deficit-focused approach "perpetuates the idea that to have a disability is to be an incomplete or broken human being" (Harmon et al., 2009, p. 137). Indeed, disabled people are often portrayed as inferior, dependent, or a burden to others (Nelson, 2000). It is essential, therefore, that diversity is celebrated rather than tolerated with the strengths associated with disability also considered

(Armstrong, 2012). Education and training initiatives should address the importance and function of workplace accommodations. For example, the benefits of providing workplace accommodations (increased productivity, employee retention, etc.) should be clearly communicated to ensure that line managers support these accommodations and non-disabled colleagues do not misinterpret workplace accommodations as an unfair advantage.

It is important to ensure that disability-oriented education and training covers a range of impairment types. As previously discussed, there appears to be a "hierarchy" of impairments, with some conditions perceived to be more legitimate or deserving of support (Freeze et al., 1999; Thomas, 2000). In particular, it is important to consider invisible conditions, which are often poorly understood or not afforded the same status as visible impairments. One of my interviewees commented: *"It would be really helpful if there was something about working with students and staff with invisible illnesses and how other people should manage and work with those students and staff, and what they, they shouldn't do, in terms of 'You don't look ill' comments and all these types of things. The do's and don'ts and just something along those lines to highlight the fact that there are people out there that you may not think are suffering with these conditions, but they are suffering. And if you knew a bit more about it, you'd understand why"* (Academic 1).

Similarly, institutions often classify employees as either fully well and able to complete all roles and responsibilities or absent due to ill health, with the notable exception of phased return following a period of long-term absence. As described by one academic, "colleagues ... assumed you were either able-bodied enough to do your job or you weren't" (Chouinard, 1995, p. 5). Another commented, "I started to improve so my GP said to [current institution] 'can she come back on a rehab scheme?' ... they said 'no', they said 'no, she's either well or she's ill, can't have somebody who's possibly ill on campus, she might be a health and safety risk'" (Williams, 2011, p. 162). Greater understanding and acceptance that there is a condition other than fully well or absent due to illness is required. This would provide greater flexibility to disabled employees, especially those with unpredictable or fluctuating conditions.

It is important that training provides a meaningful understanding of disability and is not a tokenistic approach to training that is completed as a simple tick box exercise. A real understanding of disability-related issues is required. As summarized by one interviewee: *"You've got to educate them about systemic and unconscious ableism. Because they don't know the first thing about it. And only by understanding a social model of disability, can people begin to move on and stop seeing disability in terms of a deficit model or in terms of a medical model. Or this idea of what's wrong with you all the time. The idea is well there's nothing wrong, we're just different in some regards. But the ignorance is just boundless, really. So that would be the thing, But I mean, it's a real root and branch thing that you have everybody do it. You can't just put out some kind of e-module where people spend an hour clicking their way through, you know, do they understand this term from the Equality Act, have absolutely no understanding of the framework of the concepts, of the idea of what is legal and what's not legal, and they don't care, either*" (Academic 10).

Personal accounts (e.g. Brown, 2021; Mellifont et al., 2019) provide an especially valuable insight into the challenges experienced by academics with disabilities and the measures that can support disabled faculty. For example, England (2016) provides a reflective account of her experiences as an academic with bipolar disorder. In particular, she discusses the decision to disclose the condition, a decision that she describes as both personal (facilitating support from loved ones) and political (to reduce the stigma associated with mental health conditions). She also makes a number of recommendations to faculty with bipolar disorder, including early recognition of symptoms and engagement with social support. It is important that these personal accounts are respected and listened to (Russo & Beresford, 2015). Indeed, a number of campaigns have included personal experiences to focus attention on disability in academia. These campaigns include the *Voices of Academia* social media campaign that raises the profile of mental health in higher education (https:// voicesofacademia.com/).

Individual disabled academics should not of course be compelled to represent the university or the institution's commitment to equality, diversity, and inclusion. Indeed, disabled academics often report that their advocacy work is afforded a low status or not compensated for in academic workloads. As one academic explains, disabled faculty "are not only expected to achieve 'normal' standards, amounts, ways of working but we are also expected to achieve extra in terms of disability services to the University whether by teaching or advising on estates, HR policies etc which isn't acknowledged, remunerated, nor are we really often trained for" (Williams, 2011, p. 188). Engagement in this manner may also be distressing. As summarized by another academic, "I am literally 'wheeled out' within the institution as some kind of standard bearer for the Equality Act, which was not always a comfortable experience" (Martin, 2017, p. 18).

COVID-19 and remote working

The COVID-19 pandemic has had a dramatic impact on academic practice, with both positive and negative consequences for disabled academics. In particular, there has been a transition to remote working. Teaching has been delivered online with additional activities (e.g. academic conferences and training) also adopting an online format. Online delivery has provided greater accessibility for many disabled academics and demonstrated the utility of remote working – a request that was often denied to disabled faculty prior to the pandemic. Historically, faculty have been expected to be physically present (Shelley-Egan, 2020). Indeed, academics are often expected to travel long distances for events (e.g. external examiner attendance at exam board meetings) and a full day spent travelling for a one- or two-hour meeting is not uncommon. As a consequence, those who have been unable to travel to meetings, conferences, and so on have traditionally been disadvantaged.

Physical attendance and routine commuting can, of course, be especially challenging for disabled academics. For example, travelling requires substantial energy, can interrupt medication or treatment schedules, and may require more expensive or time-consuming forms of transport. As summarized by one interviewee: *"I didn't realize how energy sapping commuting is, or working in an open plan office. I was in an open plan office with, if it was full, almost 40 people maybe 30. And that was quite tough sometimes, having the energy it takes to drown out the noise, concentrating, all of that"* (Academic 9). The COVID-19 pandemic has demonstrated that remote working is possible and created the infrastructure that is necessary to support remote working. This is of benefit not only to disabled academics but also those who have caring responsibilities. It is important, therefore, that as the risk of COVID-19 declines, we retain practices that have increased accessibility (Brown et al., 2020; Sarju, 2021).

As employers consider post lockdown practice, it is important to reflect on experience of remote working and how this can improve provision for disabled faculty. As summarized by one of my interviewees: *"People are talking about going back and whatever. But I'm like, I just don't want to have to go back to what it was, I want the flexibility, I want to be able to come in for a day or two days a week or, you know, whatever suits. On that side, I really wish we would have gotten there, though, without the pandemic. I don't know why it took this. I mean, the disabled community has been talking about this for ages"* (Academic 9). Of course, it is important to acknowledge that interest in remote working may vary. Whilst this has been valuable for some academics (e.g. providing opportunities to rest during the day), others have experienced increased isolation, anxiety, or musculoskeletal issues. Where remote working occurs, employees must have access to all required equipment and should not incur additional financial costs (e.g. printing, specialist software). Furthermore, whilst institutions may provide opportunities for staff to work from home, it is important to ensure that this does not create a "two-tier" system whereby those working from home are not provided with opportunities to network or contribute to academic discussion.

It is also important to reflect upon the disproportionate impact of the pandemic on disabled people. Though the pandemic has impacted on all sectors of the community, people with disabilities have experienced additional stressors, including increased susceptibility to COVID-19, the need for stricter isolation or shielding, reduced access to medical care, and higher levels of COVID-related mortality (e.g. Landes et al., 2020). Disability activists have also highlighted the impact of rhetoric focused on the relative value of disabled and non-disabled lives. The notion that a disabled life is less valuable than the life of a non-disabled person (whether it be in terms of the risk of infection or requiring disabled people to isolate in order to allow non-disabled people to "return to normal") reinforces stereotypical notions that disabled people are a burden to society

(Nelson, 2000). Such issues were not limited to abstract discussion, with priority afforded to the medical treatment of those without disabilities (Goggin & Ellis, 2020; Lund & Ayers, 2020; Scully, 2020). These issues clearly impact on the wellbeing of disabled academics. For example, disabled faculty may have been required to shield for lengthy periods but also in routine contact with carers. Additional issues have also been apparent. For example, some disabled academics were placed in the uncomfortable position of being required to disclose a disability for their "vulnerable" or "highly vulnerable" status to be recognized and for appropriate accommodations (e.g. remote working) to be considered (NADSN, 2020). The impact of the COVID-19 pandemic on disabled academics should not be underestimated.

Brown et al. (2020) provide a number of recommendations to improve post COVID-19 practice. For example, academics delivering online teaching during the pandemic should not be disadvantaged if their student evaluations are less favourable than when delivering their typical offline teaching. They argue that higher education institutions should use the COVID-19 pandemic experience to "ensure that any line management training, policies and procedures pertaining to managing Disabled workers ... are robustly equality impact assessed/analysed if they have not already. This will ensure they do not have a differential or adverse impact on certain groups, which are protected by law against discrimination" (Brown et al., 2020). For more information on COVID-19-related or remote working accommodations, see guidance from the National Association of Disabled Staff Networks (NADSN, 2020) and the Chronic Illness Inclusion Project (CIIP, 2020). For personal accounts of disabled academics transitioning to remote working during COVID-19, see Hannam-Swain and Bailey (2021).

Of course, many academics fear that long-term changes to academia will be inadequate. One interviewee described her experience during the pandemic and concerns that online provision will be of poorer quality than physical attendance: "*I've gone to conferences, I've gone to training days, it's been very exciting from a connectivity point of view. I'm not looking forward to the inevitable follow up, which is they decide, 'Oh, well, people don't want this any more, people are really super into meeting in person we'll just turn it all off.' I worry that once people can do things physically again, because you know there are aspects of it that are better, there'll be that push for that. And there'll be a video on but the focus won't be on it. And I just I think it will be much less good, who manages to integrate and not, like we won't have the experience of we're at a conference in breakout rooms. We'll have it but won't mix around because there'll be loads of people in physical breakout rooms, and about six people are in the special disability breakout room that they might forget to turn on and off at the right times. I think it will become more of an afterthought. And I also think there'll probably be a backlash of 'No, we don't want this, we want to have the authentic in-person experience'. So no electronics to you know, reground us*" (Academic 11). It is essential, therefore, to ensure that the quality of the online experience is maintained.

Summary

Disabled academics are systematically disadvantaged compared to their non-disabled colleagues. Universities should review current provision in order to support faculty with disabilities. There are a wealth of resources available to provide guidance and support the implementation of these recommendations. These include both personal accounts and examples of best practice (e.g. Brown, 2021; Mellifont et al., 2019).

Additional sources of interest

National Association of Disability Practitioners. The professional organization for disability practitioners. https://nadp-uk.org

National Association of Disabled Staff Networks (NADSN). An organization that connects and represents disabled staff networks. It is open to individuals and organizations. A range of resources are freely available. https://www.nadsn-uk-org

PurpleSpace. A professional networking site for disabled employees. Guidance is also provided for employers and Disability Staff Networks. https://www.purplespace.org

Voices of Academia. The site includes a range of personal accounts (blogs and podcasts) focused on mental health and wellbeing in academia. https://voicesofacademia.com

Women in Academia Support Network. A community of female researchers and podcast. https://www.wiasn.com

Conclusion

As outlined in this book, academia represents a challenging environment that is increasingly characterized by long working hours and performance management. For disabled faculty, these issues present additional challenges. For example, it is difficult for academics with energy-limiting conditions to engage in the long working hours required by the role. Despite this, there has been little consideration of disabled academics, with the majority of previous educational research focused on students with disabilities. It is clear that many disabled academics experience stigma, prejudice, and discrimination. Furthermore, the support and workplace accommodations available are not adequate. This book has been written to highlight important issues, amplify the voices and experiences of disabled faculty, and prompt changes to current practice. Without this change, academia will continue to systematically disadvantage those with disabilities.

References

Adams, S., Bekker, S., Fan, Y., Gordon, T., Shepherd, L. J., Slavich, E., & Waters, D. (2021). Gender bias in student evaluations of teaching: 'Punish[ing] those who fail to do their gender right'. *Higher Education*. https://doi.org/10.1007/s10734-021-00704-9

Alston, R. J., & Hampton, J. L. (2000). Science and Engineering as viable career choices for students with disabilities: A survey of parents and teachers. *Rehabilitation Counseling Bulletin*, *43*(3), 158–164. https://doi.org/10.1177/003435520004300306

Ameri, M., Schur, L., Adya, M., Bentley, F. S., McKay, P., & Kruse, D. (2018). The disability employment puzzle: A field experiment on employer hiring behavior. *ILR Review*, *71*(2), 329–364. https://doi.org/10.1177/0019793917717474

American Psychiatric Association (APA) (2013). *Diagnostic and statistical manual of mental disorders* (5th edition). Arlington, VA: APA.

Amtmann, D., Bamer, A. M., Cook, K. F., Askew, R. L., Noonan, V. K., & Brockway, J. A. (2012). University of Washington Self-Efficacy Scale: A new self-efficacy scale for people with disabilities. *Archives of Physical Medicine and Rehabilitation*, *93*(10), 1757–1765. https://doi.org/10.1016/j.apmr.2012.05.001

Anderson, A. (2018). Autism and the academic library: A study of online communication. *College and Research Libraries*, *79*(5), 645–658. https://doi.org/10.5860/crl.79.5.645

Anderson, R. C. (2006). Teaching (with) disability: Pedagogies of lived experience. *Review of Education, Pedagogy, and Cultural Studies*, *28*(3/4), 367–379. https://doi.org/10.1080/10714410600873258

Andersson, J., Luthra, R., Hurtig, P., & Tideman, M. (2015). Employer attitudes toward hiring persons with disabilities: A vignette study in Sweden. *Journal of Vocational Rehabilitation*, *43*(1), 41–50. https://doi.org/10.3233/JVR-150753

Angermeyer, M. C., & Schulze, B. (2001). Reducing the stigma of schizophrenia: Understanding the process and options for interventions. *Epidemiology and Psychiatric Sciences*, *10*(1), 1–7. https://doi.org/10.1017/S1121189X00008472

Anon. (2018). When I admitted I was HIV positive, my fellow academics excluded me. https://www.theguardian.com/higher-education-network/2018/may/25/when-i-admitted-i-was-hiv-positive-my-fellow-academics-excluded-me (accessed 29 August 2020).

Arbuckle, J., & Williams, R. D. (2003). Students' perceptions of expressiveness: Age and gender effects on teacher evaluations. *Sex Roles*, *49*(9), 507–516. https://doi.org/10.1023/A.1025832707002

Armitage, R., & Nellums, L. B. (2020). The COVID-19 response must be disability inclusive. *Lancet Public Health*, *5*(5), e257. https://doi.org/10.1016/S2468-2667(20)30076-1

Armstrong, T. (2012). First, discover their strengths. *Educational Leadership*, *70*(2), 10–16. https://www.ascd.org/el/articles/first-discover-their-strengths (accessed 11 January 2021).

Arnold, L. M., Crofford, L. J., Mease, P. J., Burgess, S. M., Palmer, S. C., Abetz, L., & Martin, S. A. (2008). Patient perspectives on the impact of fibromyalgia. *Patient Education and Counseling*, *73*(1), 114–120. https://doi.org/10.1016/j.pec.2008.06.005

Arthur, L. (2009). From performativity to professionalism: Lecturers' responses to student feedback. *Teaching in Higher Education*, *14*(4), 441–454. https://doi.org/10.1080/13562510903050228

References 107

Baldridge, D. C., & Veiga, J. F. (2001). Toward a greater understanding of the willingness to request an accommodation: Can requesters' beliefs disable the Americans with Disabilities Act? *Academy of Management Review, 26*(1), 85–99. https://doi.org/10.5465/amr.2001.4011956

Baldwin, R. G., & Wawrzynski, M. R. (2011). Contingent faculty as teachers: What we know; what we need to know. *American Behavioral Scientist, 55*(11), 1485–1509. https://doi.org/10.1177/0002764211409194

Ball, S. J. (2012). Performativity, commodification and commitment: An I-Spy guide to the neoliberal university. *British Journal of Education Studies, 60*(1), 17–28. https://doi.org/10.1080/00071005.2011.650940

Ballard, S. L., Bartle, E., & Masequesmay, G. (2008). *Finding queer allies: The impact of ally training and safe zone stickers on campus climate.* https://files.eric.ed.gov/fulltext/ED517219.pdf (accessed 11 January 2021).

Balser, D. B. (2007). Predictors of workplace accommodations for employees with mobility-related disabilities. *Administration and Society, 39*(5), 656–683. https://doi.org/10.1177/0095399707303639

Battye, L. (1966) The Chatterley syndrome. In P. Hunt (ed.) *Stigma: The experience of disability* (pp. 3–16). London: Geoffrey Chapman.

Beacom, A., French, L., & Kendall, S. (2016). Reframing impairment: Continuity and change in media representations of disability through the Paralympic Games. *International Journal of Sport Communication, 9*(1), 42–62. https://doi.org/10.1123/ijsc.2015-0077

Beam, S. N., & Clay-Buck, H. (2018). Low-spoon teaching: Labor, gender, and self-accommodation in academia. *Tulsa Studies in Women's Literature, 37*(1), 173–180. https://doi.org/10.1353/tsw.2018.0008

Beasley, B. W., Simon, S. D., & Wright, S. M. (2006). A time to be promoted: The prospective study of promotion in academia. *Journal of General Internal Medicine, 21*(2), 123–129. https://doi.org/10.1111/j.1525-1497.2005.00297.x

Beatty, J. (2001). *Chronic illness identity in the workplace.* Academy of Management Conference, Washington, August.

Beyerbach, B. (2005). The social foundations classroom: Themes in sixty years of teachers in film: Fast Times, Dangerous Minds, Stand on Me. *Educational Studies, 37*(3), 267–285. https://doi.org/10.1207/s15326993es3703_5

Bezin, J., Francis, F., Nguyen, N. V., Robinson, P., Blin, P., Fourrier-Reglat, A., Pariente, A., & Moore, N. (2017). Impact of a public media event on the use of statins in the French population. *Archives of Cardiovascular Disease, 110*(2), 91–98. https://doi.org/10.1016/j.acvd.2016.05.002

Bianchini, K. J., Greve, K. W., & Glynn, G. (2005). On the diagnosis of malingered pain-related disability: Lessons from cognitive malingering research. *The Spine Journal, 5*(4), 404–417. https://doi.org/10.1016/j.spinee.2004.11.016

Bilimoria, D., & Stewart, A. J. (2009). 'Don't ask, don't tell': The academic climate for lesbian, gay, bisexual, and transgender faculty in Science and Engineering. *NWSA Journal, 21*(2), 85–103.

Blanck, P. (2011). Disability and aging: Historical and contemporary views. In R. L. Wiener & S. L. Willborn (eds.) *Disability and aging discrimination: Perspectives in law and psychology* (pp. 49–70). New York: Springer.

Bloch, C., Graversen, E. K., & Pedersen, H. S. (2014). Competitive research grants and their impact on career performance. *Minerva, 52*(1), 77–96. https://doi.org/10.1007/s11024-014-9247-0

Bogart, K. R. (2014). The role of disability self-concept in adaptation to congenital or acquired disability. *Rehabilitation Psychology, 59*(1), 107–115. https://doi.org/1037/a0035800

References

Boswell, S. S. (2016). Ratemyprofessors is hogwash (but I care): Effects of Ratemyprofessors and university-administered teaching evaluations on professors. *Computers in Human Behavior, 56*, 155–162. https://doi.org/10.1016/j.chb.2015.11.045

Bouziri, H., Smith, D. R. M., Descatha, A., Dab, W., & Jean, K. (2020). Working from home in the time of COVID-19: How to best preserve occupational health. *Occupational and Environmental Medicine, 77*(7), 509–510. https://doi.org/10.1136/oemed-2020-106599

Boyd, K., Woodbury-Smith, M., & Szatmari, P. (2011). Managing anxiety and depressive symptoms in adults with autism spectrum disorders. *Journal of Psychiatry and Neuroscience, 36*(4), E35–E36. https://doi.org/10.1503/jpn.110040

Bozzon, R., Murgia, A., Poggio, B., & Rapetti, E. (2017). Work–life interferences in the early stages of academic careers: The case of precarious researchers in Italy. *European Educational Research Journal, 16*(2/3), 332–351. https://doi.org/10.1177/1474904116669364

Braun, D. C., Gormally, C., & Clark, M. D. (2017). The Deaf Mentoring Survey: A community cultural wealth framework for measuring mentoring effectiveness with underrepresented students. *CBE: Life Sciences Education, 16*, 10. https://doi.org/10.1187/cbe.15-07.0155

Briant, E., Watson, N., & Philo, G. (2013). Reporting disability in the age of austerity: The changing face of media representation of disability and disabled people in the United Kingdom and the creation of new 'folk devils'. *Disability and Society, 28*(6), 874–889. https://doi.org/10.1080/09687599.2013.813837

Bridges, D. (2011). Research quality assessment: Intended and unintended consequences. *Power and Education, 3*(1), 31–38. https://doi.org/10.2304/power.2011.3.1.31

Brisenden, S. (1986). Independent living and the medical model of disability. *Disability, Handicap and Society, 1*(2), 173–178. https://doi.org/10.1080/02674648666780171

Brown, N. (2021). *Lived experiences of ableism in academia: Strategies for inclusion in higher education*. Bristol: Policy Press.

Brown, N., & Leigh, J. (2018). Ableism in academia: Where are the disabled and ill academics? *Disability and Society, 33*(6), 985–989. https://doi.org/10.1080/09687599.2018.1455627

Brown, N., & Leigh, J. (2020). *Ableism in academia: Theorising experiences of disabilities and chronic illnesses in higher education*. London: UCL Press.

Brown, N., Nicholson, J., Campbell, F. K., Patel, M., Knight, R., & Moore, S. (2020). COVID-19 post-lockdown: Perspectives, implications and strategies for disabled staff. *Alter, 15*(3), 262–269. https://doi.org/10.1016/j.alter.2020.12.005

Brown, N., Thompson, P., & Leigh, J. S. (2018). Making academia more accessible. *Journal of Perspectives in Applied Academic Practice, 6*(2). https://doi.org/10.14297/jpaap.v6i2.348

Brown Johnson, C. G., Brodsky, J. L., & Cataldo, J. K. (2014). Lung cancer stigma, anxiety, depression, and quality of life. *Journal of Psychosocial Oncology, 32*(1), 59–73. https://doi.org/10.1080/07347332.2013.855963

Budge, F., Schippers, A., Kool, J., Miranda-Galarza, B., & van Hove, G. (2016). More than a 'nice day out': How to encourage the meaningful participation of people with learning difficulties in disability conferences. *Sky Journal of Educational Research, 4*(3), 27–34. http://www.skyjournals.org/sjer/abstract/2016/May/Budge%20et%20al.htm (accessed 11 January 2021).

Burgstahler, S., & Doe, T. (2004). Disability-related simulations: If, when, and how to use them in professional development. *Review of Disability Studies, 1*(2), 8–18. https://www.rdsjournal.org/index.php/journal/article/view/385 (accessed 11 January 2021).

Burns, E., Poikkeus, A. M., & Aro, M. (2013). Resilience strategies employed by teachers with dyslexia working at tertiary education. *Teaching and Teacher Education, 34*, 77–85. https://doi.org/10.1016/j.tate.2013.04.007

Cahill, S. E., & Eggleston, R. (1995). Reconsidering the stigma of physical disability: Wheelchair use and public kindness. *Sociological Quarterly*, *36*(4), 681–698. https://doi.org/10.1111/j.1533-8525.1995.tb00460.x

Cai, R. Y., & Richdale, A. L. (2016). Educational experiences and needs of higher education students with autism spectrum disorder. *Journal of Autism and Developmental Disorders*, *46*(1), 31–41. https://doi.org/10.1007/s10803-015-2535-1

Callus, A. M. (2017). Making disability conferences more actively inclusive. *Disability and Society*, *32*(10), 1661–1665. https://doi.org/10.1080/09687599.2017.1356059

Cameron, H. E. (2016). Beyond cognitive deficit: The everyday lived experience of dyslexic students at university. *Disability and Society*, *31*(2), 223–239. https://doi.org/10.1080/09687599.2016.1152951

Campbell, E. (2018). Reconstructing my identity: An autoethnographic exploration of depression and anxiety in academia. *Journal of Organizational Ethnography*, *7*(3), 235–246. https://doi.org/10.1108/JOE-10-2017-0045

Cannizzo, F., Mauri, C., & Osbaldiston, N. (2019). Moral barriers between work/life balance policy and practice in academia. *Journal of Cultural Economy*, *12*(4), 251–264. https://doi.org/10.1080/17530350.2019.1605400

Cardel, M. I., Dean, N., & Montoya-Williams, D. (2020). Preventing a secondary epidemic of lost early career scientists: Effects of COVID-19 pandemic on women with children. *Annals of the American Thoracic Society*, *17*(11), 1366–1370. https://doi.org/10.1513/AnnalsATS.202006-589IP

Cardoso, J. P., Ribeiro, I. Q. B., de Araujo, T. M., & dos Reis, E. J. F. B. (2009). Prevalence of musculoskeletal pain among teachers. *Revista Brasileira de Epidemiologia*, *12*(4), 1–10. https://www.scielosp.org/pdf/rbepid/2009.v12n4/604-614/en (accessed 11 January 2021).

Carr, S. (2019). 'I am not your nutter': A personal reflection on commodification and comradeship in service user and survivor research. *Disability and Society*, *34*(7), 1140–1153. https://doi.org/10.1080/09687599.2019.1608424

Carusi, F. T., Di Paolantonio, M., Hodgson, N., & Ramaekers, S. (2020). Doing academia in "COVID-19 times". *Antistasis*, *10*(3). https://journals.lib.unb.ca/index.php/antistasis/article/view/31440 (accessed 11 January 2021).

Castellacci, F., & Vinas-Bardolet, C. (2020). Permanent contracts and job satisfaction: Evidence from European countries. *Studies in Higher Education*, *46*(9), 1866–1880. https://doi.org/10.1080/03075079.2019.1711041

Caton, S., & Chapman, M. (2016). The use of social media and people with intellectual disability: A systematic review and thematic analysis. *Journal of Intellectual and Developmental Disability*, *41*(2), 125–139. https://doi.org/10.3109/13668250.2016.1153052

Chapple, A., Ziebland, S., & McPherson, A. (2004). Stigma, shame, and blame experienced by patients with lung cancer: Qualitative study. *British Medical Journal*, *328*(7454), 1470. https://doi.org/10.1136/bmj.38111.639734.7C

Charmaz, K. (1991). *Good days, bad days: The self in chronic illness and time*. New Brunswick, NJ: Rutgers University Press.

Chen, M., & Lawrie, S. (2017). Newspaper depictions of mental and physical health. *BJPsych Bulletin*, *41*(6), 308–313. https://doi.org/10.1192/pb.bp.116.054775

Cheng, H. Y. K., Wong, M. T., Yu, Y. C., & Ju, Y. Y. (2016). Work-related musculoskeletal disorders and ergonomic risk factors in special education teachers and teacher's aides. *BMC Public Health*, *16*(1), 137. https://doi.org/10.1186/s12889-016-2777-7

Chiang, E. S. (2020). Disability cultural centers: How colleges can move beyond access to inclusion. *Disability and Society*, *35*(7), 1183–1188. https://doi.org/10.1080/09687599.2019.1679536

Chouinard, V. (1995). Like Alice through the looking glass: Accommodation in academia. *Resources for Feminist Research*, *24*(3/4), 3–11.

Choy, E., Perrot, S., Leon, T., Kaplan, J., Petersel, D., Ginovker, A., & Kramer, E. (2010). A patient survey of the impact of fibromyalgia and the journey to diagnosis. *BMC Health Services Research, 10*, 102. https://doi.org/10.1186/1472-6963-10-102

Chronic Illness Inclusion Project (CIIP) (2020). *Turning the remote access revolution into reasonable adjustments: Guidance on including disabled people in face-to-face meetings using videoconferencing technology.* https://www.centreforwelfarereform.org/uploads/attachment/747/remote-revolution-to-reasonable-adjustments.pdf

Chu, L. F., Utengen, A., Kadry, B., Kucharski, S. E., Campos, H., Crockett, J., Dawson, N., & Clauson, K. A. (2016). 'Nothing about us without us': Patient partnership in medical conferences. *British Medical Journal, 354*, i3883. https://doi.org/10.1136/bmj.i3883

Clair, J. A., Beatty, J. E., & McLean, T. L. (2005). Out of sight but not out of mind: Managing invisible social identities in the workplace. *Academy of Management Review, 30*(1), 78–95. https://doi.org/10.5465/amr.2005.15281431

Clegg, C., Fremouw, W., & Mogge, N. (2009). Utility of the Structured Inventory of Malingered Symptomology (SIMS) and the Assessment of Depression Inventory (ADI) in screening for malingering among outpatients seeking to claim disability. *Journal of Forensic Psychiatry and Psychology, 20*(2), 239–254. https://doi.org/10.1080/14789940802267760

Clement, S., Lassman, F., Barley, E., Evans-Lacko, S., Williams, P., Yamaguchi, S., Slade, M., Rusch, N., & Thornicroft, G. (2013). Mass media interventions for reducing mental health-related stigma. *Cochrane Database of Systematic Reviews, 7*, CD009453. https://doi.org/10.1002/14651858.CD009453.pub2

Clément-Guillotin, C., Rohmer, O., Forestier, C., Guillotin, P., Deshayes, M., & d'Arripe-Longueville, F. (2018). Implicit and explicit stereotype content associated with people with physical disability: Does sport change anything? *Psychology of Sport and Exercise, 38*, 192–201. https://doi.org/10.1016/j.psychsport.2018.06.014

Cohen, J., Schiffler, F., Rohmer, O., Louvet, E., & Mollaret, P. (2019). Is disability really an obstacle to success? Impact of a disability simulation on motivation and performance. *Journal of Applied Social Psychology, 49*, 50–59. https://doi.org/10.1111/jasp.12564

Colella, A. (2001). Coworker distributive fairness judgments of the workplace accommodation of employees with disabilities. *Academy of Management Review, 26*(1), 100–116. https://doi.org/10.5465/amr.2001.4011984

Collins, M. E., & Mowbray, C. T. (2005). Higher education and psychiatric disabilities: National survey of campus disability services. *American Journal of Orthopsychiatry, 75*(2), 304–315. https://doi.org/10.1037/0002-9432.75.2.304

Collins, N. L., & Miller, L. C. (1994). Self-disclosure and liking: A meta-analytic review. *Psychological Bulletin, 116*(3), 457–475. https://doi.org/10.1037/0033-2909.116.3.457

Collinson, C., & Penketh, C. (2010). 'Sit in the corner and don't eat the crayons': Postgraduates with dyslexia and the dominant 'lexic' discourse. *Disability and Society, 25*(1), 7–19. https://doi.org/10.1080/09687590903363274

Copeland, J., Chan, F., Bezyak, J., & Fraser, R. T. (2010). Assessing cognitive and affective reactions of employers toward people with disabilities in the workplace. *Journal of Occupational Rehabilitation, 20*(4), 427–434. https://doi.org/10.1007/s10926-009-9207-y

Corbera, E., Anguelovski, I., Honey-Roses, J., & Ruiz-Mallen, I. (2020). Academia in the time of COVID-19: Towards an ethics of care. *Planning, Theory and Practice, 21*(2), 191–199. https://doi.org/10.1080/14649357.2020.1757891

Costa, A. J., Labuda Schrop, S., McCord, G., & Ritter, C. (2005). Depression in family medicine faculty. *Family Medicine, 37*(4), 271–275. https://pubmed.ncbi.nlm.nih.gov/15812697/ (accessed 11 January 2021).

Crompton, E. (2017). Why schizophrenia need not rob us of a life in academia. https://www.theguardian.com/higher-education-network/2017/feb/01/schizophrenia-successful-academic-career-mental-health (accessed 29 August 2020).

Crook, S. (2020). Parenting during the COVID-19 pandemic of 2020: Academia, labour and care work. *Women's History Review, 29*(7), 1226–1238. https://doi.org/10.1080/09612025.2020.1807690

Crow, L. (1996). Including all our lives: Renewing the social model of disability. In J. Morris (ed.) *Encounters with strangers: Feminism and disability*. London: Women's Press.

Currie, J., & Eveline, J. (2011). E-technology and work/life balance for academics with young children. *Higher Education, 62*, 533–550. https://doi.org/10.1007/s10734-010-9404-9

Davies, S. W., Putnam, H. M., Ainsworth, T., Baum, J. K., Bove, C. B., Crosby, S. C., … Bates, A.E. (2021). Promoting inclusive metrics of success and impact to dismantle a discriminatory reward system in science. *PLoS Biology, 19*(6), e3001282. https://doi.org/10.1371/journal.pbio.3001282

De Picker, M. (2020). Rethinking inclusion and disability activism at academic conferences: Strategies proposed by a PhD student with a physical disability. *Disability and Society, 35*(1), 163–167. https://doi.org/10.1080/09687599.2019.1619234

Deal, M. (2006). *Attitudes of disabled people toward other disabled people and impairment groups*. Unpublished doctoral thesis, City University, London. https://openaccess.city.ac.uk/17416/

Delucchi, M., & Korgen, K. (2002). 'We're the customer: We pay the tuition': Student consumerism among undergraduate sociology majors. *Teaching Sociology, 30*(1), 100–107. https://doi.org/10.2307/3211524

DePauw, K. P. (1997). The (In)Visibility of DisAbility: Cultural contexts and 'sporting bodies'. *Quest, 49*(4), 416–430. https://doi.org/10.1080/00336297.1997.10484258

de Wolfe, P. (2009). ME: The rise and fall of media sensation. *Medical Sociology Online, 4*(1), 2–13.

Dickerson, F. B., Sommerville, J., Origoni, A. E., Ringel, N. B., & Parente, F. (2002). Experiences of stigma among outpatients with schizophrenia. *Schizophrenia Bulletin, 28*(1), 143–155. https://doi.org/10.1093/oxfordjournals.schbul.a006917

Diefenbach, D. L., & West, M. D. (2007). Television and attitudes toward mental health issues: Cultivation analysis and the third-person effect. *Journal of Community Psychology, 35*(2), 181–195. https://doi.org/10.1002/jcop.20142

Dobele, A. R., & Rundle-Theile, S. (2015). Progression through academic ranks: A longitudinal examination of internal promotion drivers. *Higher Education Quarterly, 69*(4), 410–429. https://doi.org/10.1111/hequ.12081

Dolmage, J. (2015). Universal Design: Places to start. *Disability Studies Quarterly, 35*(2). https://doi.org/10.18061/dsq.v35i2.4632

Dorfman, D. (2019). Fear of the disability con: Perceptions of fraud and special rights discourse. *Law and Society Review, 53*(4), 1051–1091. https://doi.org/10.1111/lasr.12437

Dozier, R. (2015). A view from the academe: Lesbian and gay faculty and minority stress. *Psychology of Sexual Orientation and Gender Diversity, 2*(2), 188–198. https://doi.org/10.1037/sgd0000105

Draper, W. R., Reid, C. A., & McMahon, B. T. (2011). Workplace discrimination and the perception of disability. *Rehabilitation Counseling Bulletin, 55*(1), 29–37. https://doi.org/10.1177/0034355210392792

Edwards, C., & Harold, G. (2014). DeafSpace and the principles of Universal Design. *Disability and Rehabilitation, 36*, 1350–1359. https://doi.org/10.3109/09638288.2014.913710

England, M. R. (2016). Being open in academia: A personal narrative of mental illness and disclosure. *Canadian Geographer, 60*(2), 226–231. https://doi.org/10.1111/cag.12270

Entman, R. M. (2007). Framing bias: Media in the distribution of power. *Journal of Communication, 57*(1), 163–173. https://doi.org/10.1111/j.1460-2466.2006.00336.x

Erick, P. N., & Smith, D. R. (2011). A systematic review of musculoskeletal disorders among school teachers. *BMC Musculoskeletal Disorders, 12*(260). https://doi.org/10.1186/1471-2474-12-260

Evans, H. D. (2019). 'Trial by fire': Forms of impairment disclosure and implications for disability identity. *Disability and Society, 34*(5), 726–746. https://doi.org/10.1080/09687599.2019.1580187

Evans, W. (2014). 'If they can't tell the difference between duphalac and digoxin you've got patient safety issues'. Nurse lecturers' constructions of students' dyslexic identities in nurse education. *Nurse Education Today, 34*(6), e41–e46. https://doi.org/10.1016/j.nedt.2013.11.004

Fan, Y., Shepherd, L. J., Slavich, E., Waters, D., Stone, M., Abel, R., & Johnston, E. L. (2019). Gender and cultural bias in student evaluations: Why representation matters. *PLoS ONE, 14*(2), e0209749. https://doi.org/10.1371/journal.pone.0209749

Felton, J., Koper, P. T., Mitchell, J., & Stinson, M. (2008). Attractiveness, easiness and other issues: Student evaluations of professors on Ratemyprofessors.com. *Assessment and Evaluation in Higher Education, 33*(1), 45–61. https://doi.org/10.1080/02602930601122803

Files, J. A., Mayer, A. P., Ko, M. G., Friedrich, P., Jenkins, M., Bryan, M. J., ... & Hayes, S. N. (2017). Speaker introductions at internal medicine grand rounds: Forms of address reveal gender bias. *Journal of Women's Health, 26*(5), 413–419. https://doi.org/10.1089/jwh.2016.6044

Finkelstein, V. (1980). *Attitudes and disabled people: Issues for discussion*. Monograph #5. New York: World Rehabilitation Fund.

Fischer, J., Ritchie, E. G., & Hanspach, J. (2012). Academia's obsession with quantity. *Trends in Ecology and Evolution, 27*(9), 473–474. https://doi.org/10.1016/j.tree.2012.05.010

Fishbain, D. A., Cutler, R., Rosomoff, H. L., & Rosomoff, R. S. (1999). Chronic pain disability: Exaggeration/malingering and submaximal effort research. *Clinical Journal of Pain, 15*(4), 244–274. https://doi.org/10.1097/00002508-199912000-00002

Fitzgerald, M. H., & Paterson, K. A. (1995). The hidden disability dilemma for the preservation of self. *Journal of Occupational Science, 2*(1), 13–21. https://doi.org/10.1080/14427591.1995.9686392

Fjellman-Wiklund, A., & Sundelin, G. (1998). Musculoskeletal discomfort of music teachers: An eight-year perspective and psychological work factors. *International Journal of Occupational and Environmental Health, 4*(2), 89–98. https://doi.org/10.1179/oeh.1998.4.2.89

Flower, A., Burns, M. K., & Bottsford-Miller, N. A. (2007). Meta-analysis of disability simulation research. *Remedial and Special Education, 28*(2), 72–79. https://doi.org/10.1177/07419325070280020601

Foster, D. (2007). Legal obligation or personal lottery? Employee experiences of disability and the negotiation of adjustments in the public sector workplace. *Work, Employment and Society, 21*(1), 67–84. https://doi.org/10.1177/0950017007073616

Freedman, R. I., & Fesko, S. L. (1996). The meaning of work in the lives of people with significant disabilities: Consumer and family perspectives. *Journal of Rehabilitation, 62*(3), 49–55.

Freeze, R., Kueneman, R., Frankel, S., Mahon, M., & Nielsen, T. (1999). Passages to employment. *International Journal of Practical Approaches to Disability, 23*(3), 3–13.

French, S. (1988). Experiences of disabled health and caring professionals. *Sociology of Health and Illness, 10*(2), 170–188. https://doi.org/10.1111/1467-9566.ep11339941

French, S. (1992). Simulation exercises in disability awareness training: A critique. *Disability, Handicap and Society, 7*(3), 257–266. https://doi.org/10.1080/02674649266780261

Fung, K. M. T., Tsang, H. W. H., & Corrigan, P. W. (2008). Self-stigma of people with schizophrenia as predictor of their adherence to psychosocial treatment. *Psychiatric Rehabilitation Journal, 32*(2), 95–104. https://doi.org/10.2975/32.2.2008.95.104

Gallager, H. G. (1990). *By trust betrayed: Patients and physicians in the Third Reich*. London: Henry Hold.

Gardiner, M., Tiggemann, M., Kearns, H., & Marshall, K. (2007). Show me the money! An empirical analysis of mentoring outcomes for women in academia. *Higher Education Research and Development, 26*(4), 425–442. https://doi.org/10.1080/07294360701658633

Geertz, C. (1973). *The interpretation of cultures*. New York: Basic Books.

Gelbar, N. W., Shefcyk, A., & Reichow, B. (2015). A comprehensive survey of current and former college students with autism spectrum disorders. *Yale Journal of Biology and Medicine, 88*(1), 45–68. https://www.ncbi.nlm.nih.gov/pmc/articles/PMC4345538/ (accessed 11 January 2021).

Geng-quing, C., & Qu, H. (2005). A study of differential employers' attitude towards hiring people with physical, mental, and sensory disabilities in restaurant industry. *Journal of Human Resources in Hospitality and Tourism, 3*(2), 1–31. https://doi.org/10.1300/J171v03n0201

Gilbride, D., Stensrud, R., Ehlers, C., Evans, E., & Peterson, C. (2000). Employers' attitudes toward hiring persons with disabilities. *Journal of Rehabilitation, 66*(4), 17–23.

Giroux, H. A. (2014). *Neoliberalism's war on higher education*. Chicago, IL: Haymarket Books.

Giroux, H. A. (2015). *Education and the crisis of public values: Challenging the assault on teachers, students, and public education* (2nd edition). New York: Peter Lang.

Glazzard, J., & Dale, K. (2013). Trainee teachers with dyslexia: Personal narratives of resilience. *Journal of Research in Special Educational Needs, 13*(1), 26–37. https://doi.org/10.1111/j.1471-3802.2012.01254.x

Gobbo, K., & Shmulsky, S. (2014). Faculty experience with college students with autism spectrum disorders: A qualitative study of challenges and solutions. *Focus on Autism and Other Developmental Disabilities, 29*(1), 13–22. https://doi.org/10.1177/1088357613504989

Goffman, E. (1963). *Stigma: Notes on the management of spoiled identity*. New York: Simon & Schuster.

Goggin, G., & Ellis, K. (2020). Disability, communication, and life itself in the COVID-19 pandemic. *Health Sociology Review, 29*(2), 168–176. https://doi.org/10.1080/14461242.2020.1784020

Gold, P. B., Oire, S. N., Fabian, E. S., & Wewiorski, N. J. (2012). Negotiating reasonable workplace accommodations: Perspectives of employers, employees with disabilities, and rehabilitation service providers. *Journal of Vocational Rehabilitation, 37*(1), 25–37. https://doi.org/10.3233/JVR-2012-0597

Gradel, K., & Edson, A. J. (2009). Putting Universal Design for Learning on the higher ed agenda. *Journal of Educational Technology Systems, 38*(2), 111–121. https://doi.org/10.2190/ET.38.2.d

Grayson, E., & Marini, I. (1996). Simulated disability exercises and their impact on attitudes toward persons with disabilities. *International Journal of Rehabilitation Research, 19*(2), 123–131. https://doi.org/10.1097/00004356-199606000-00003

Grewal, I., Joy, S., Lewis, J., Swales, K., & Woodfield, K. (2002). *Disabled for life? Attitudes towards, and experiences of disability in Britain*. Leeds: Corporate Document Services.

Hadfield, R., Mardon, H., Barlow, D., & Kennedy, S. (1996). Delay in the diagnosis of endometriosis: A survey of women from the USA and the UK. *Human Reproduction, 11*(4), 878–880. https://doi.org/10.1093/oxfordjournals.humrep.a019270

Hall, T., & Healey, M. (2005). Disabled students' experiences of fieldwork. *Area, 37*(4), 446–449. https://doi.org/10.1111/j.1475-4762.2005.00649.x

Hallam, A. (2002). Media influences on mental health policy: Long-term effects of the Clunis and Silcock cases. *International Review of Psychiatry, 14*(1), 26–33. https://doi.org/10.1080/09540260120114032

Haller, B. A. (2010). *Representing disability in an ableist work: Essays on mass media*. Louisville, KY: The Advocado Press.

Haller, B., & Ralph, S. (2001). Profitability, diversity, and disability images in advertising in the United States and Great Britain. *Disability Studies Quarterly, 21*(2). https://doi.org/10.18061/dsq.v21i2.276

Haller, B. A., & Ralph, S. (2006). Are disability images in advertising becoming bold and daring? An analysis of prominent themes in US and UK campaigns. *Disability Studies Quarterly, 26*(3). https://doi.org/10.18061/dsq.v26i3.716

Hannam-Swain, S. (2018). The additional labour of a disabled PhD student. *Disability and Society, 33*(1), 138–142. https://doi.org/10.1080/09687599.2017.1375698

Hannam-Swain, S., & Bailey, C. (2021). Considering COVID-19: Autoethnographic practices in a time of crisis by two disabled UK academics. *Social Sciences and Humanities Open, 4*, 100145. https://doi.org/10.1016/j.ssaho.2021.100145

Hardy, A., McDonald, J., Guijt, R., Leane, E., Martin, A., James, A., Jones, M., Corban, M., & Green, B. (2018). Academic parenting: Work–family conflict and strategies across child age, disciplines and career level. *Studies in Higher Education, 43*(4), 625–643. https://doi.org/10.1080/03075079.2016.1185777

Harmon, C., Kasa-Hendrickson, C., & Neal, L. V. I. (2009). Promoting cultural competencies for teachers of students with significant disabilities. *Research and Practice for Persons with Severe Disabilities, 34*(3/4), 137–144. https://doi.org/10.2511/rpsd.34.3-4.137

Harrison, A. G., Edwards, M. J., & Parker, K. C. H. (2007). Identifying students faking ADHD: Preliminary findings and strategies for detection. *Archives of Clinical Neuropsychology, 22*(5), 577–588. https://doi.org/10.1016/j.acn.2007.03.008

Hartnett, H. P., Stuart, H., Thurman, H., Loy, B., & Batiste, L. C. (2011). Employers' perceptions of the benefits of workplace accommodations: Reasons to hire, retain and promote people with disabilities. *Journal of Vocational Rehabilitation, 34*(1), 17–23. https://doi.org/10.3233/JVR-2010-0530

Harutunian, K., Gargallo Albiol, J., Barbosa de Figueiredo, R. P., & Gay Escoda, C. (2011). Ergonomics and musculoskeletal pain among postgraduate students and faculty members of the School of Dentistry of the University of Barcelona (Spain): A cross-sectional study. *Medicina Oral Patologia Oral y Cirugia Bucal, 16*(3), e425–e429. https://doi.org/10.4317/medoral.16.e425

Harvey, D. (2005). *A brief history of Neoliberalism*. Oxford: Oxford University Press.

Hawkins, R., Manzi, M., & Ojeda, D. (2014). Lives in the making: Power, academia and the everyday. *ACME, 13*(2), 328–351. https://acme-journal.org/index.php/acme/article/view/1010 (accessed 11 January 2021).

Hayashi, R., & May, G. E. (2011). The effect of exposure to a professor with a visible disability on students' attitudes toward disabilities. *Journal of Social Work in Disability and Rehabilitation, 10*(1), 36–48. https://doi.org/10.1080/1536710X.2011.546300

Hayter, M., & Jackson, D. (2020). Pre-registration undergraduate nurses and the COVID-19 pandemic: Students or workers? *Journal of Clinical Nursing, 29*, 3115–3116. https://doi.org/10.1111/jocn.15317

Heffernan, T. (2021). Sexism, racism, prejudice, and bias: A literature review and synthesis of research surrounding student evaluations of courses and teaching. *Assessment and Evaluation in Higher Education.* https://doi.org/10.1080/02602938.2021.1888075

Heilman, R. B. (1991). The great-teacher myth. *American Scholar, 60*(3), 417–423.

Herbert, J. T. (2000). Simulation as a learning method to facilitate disability awareness. *Journal of Experiential Education, 23*(1), 5–11. https://doi.org/10.1177/105382590002300102

Herek, G. M. (1996). Why tell if you are not asked? Self-disclosure, intergroup contact, and heterosexuals' attitudes towards lesbians and gay men. In G. M. Herek, J. B. Jobe, & R. M. Carney (eds.) *Out in force: Sexual orientation and the military* (pp. 197–225). Chicago, IL: University of Chicago Press.

Hernandez, B., Keys, C., & Balcazar, F. (2000). Employer attitudes toward workers with disabilities and their ADA employment rights: A literature review. *Journal of Rehabilitation, 66*(4), 4–16.

Hewlett, S., Chalder, T., Choy, E., Cramp, F., Davis, B., Dures, E., Nicholls, C., & Kirwan, J. (2011). Fatigue in rheumatoid arthritis: Time for a conceptual model. *Rheumatology, 50*(6), 1004–1006. https://doi.org/10.1093/rheumatology/keq282

Hinds, K., & Sutcliffe, K. (2019). Heterodox and orthodox discourses in the case of Lyme disease: A synthesis of arguments. *Qualitative Health Research, 29*(11), 1661–1673. https://doi.org/10.1177/1049732319846170

Hodge, N. (2014). Unruly bodies at conference. *Disability and Society, 29*(4), 655–658. https://doi.org/10.1080/09687599.2014.894749

Holland, C., Lorenzi, F., & Hall, T. (2016). Performance anxiety in academia: Tensions within research assessment exercises in an age of austerity. *Policy Futures in Education, 14*(8), 1101–1116. https://doi.org/10.1177/1478210316664263

Holmes, G., & McElwee, G. (1995). Total quality management in higher education: How to approach human resource management. *TQM Magazine, 7*(6), 5–10. https://doi.org/10.1108/09544789510103699

Holzemer, W. L., Human, S., Arudo, J., Rosa, M. E., Hamilton, M. J., Corless, I., … & Maryland, M. (2009). Exploring HIV stigma and quality of life for persons living with HIV infection. *Journal of the Association of Nurses in AIDS Care, 20*(3), 161–168. https://doi.org/10.1016/j.jana.2009.02.002

Hopwood, C. J., Orlando, M., & Clark, T. S. (2010). The detection of malingered pain-related disability with the Personality Assessment Inventory. *Rehabilitation Psychology, 55*(3), 307–310. https://doi.org/10.1037/a0020516

Houston, D., Meyer, L. H., & Paewai, S. (2006). Academic staff workloads and job satisfaction: Expectations and values in academe. *Journal of Higher Education Policy and Management, 28*(1), 17–30. https://doi.org/10.1080/13600800500283734

Hughes, B. (2009). Wounded/monstrous/abject: A critique of the disabled body in the sociological imaginary. *Disability and Society, 24*(4), 399–410. https://doi.org/10.1080/09687590902876144

Inckle, K. (2018). Unreasonable adjustments: The additional unpaid labour of academics with disabilities. *Disability and Society, 33*(8), 1372-1376. https://doi.org/10.1080/09687599.2018.1480263

Jago, B. J. (2002). Chronicling an academic depression. *Journal of Contemporary Ethnography, 31*(6), 729–757. https://doi.org/10.1177/089124102237823

Jalali, M., Shahabi, S., Lankarani, K. B., Kamali, M., & Moigani, P. (2020). COVID-19 and disabled people: Perspectives from Iran. *Disability and Society, 35*(5), 844–847. https://doi.org/10.1080/09687599.2020.1754165

Jennings, K. S., Cheung, J. H., Britt, T. W., Goguen, K. N., Jeffirs, S. M., Peasley, A. L., & Lee, A. C. (2015). How are perceived stigma, self-stigma, and self-reliance related to treatment-seeking? A three-path model. *Psychiatric Rehabilitation Journal, 38*(2), 109–116. https://doi.org/10.1037/prj0000138

Jones, E. E., Farina, A., Hastorf, A. H., Markus, H., Miller, D. T., & Scott, R. A. (1984). *Social stigma: The psychology of marked relationships.* New York: W.H. Freeman.

Jones, G. E. (1997). Advancement opportunity issues for persons with disabilities. *Human Resource Management Review, 7*(1), 55–76. https://doi.org/10.1016/S1053-4822(97)90005-X

Jones, J., Gaffney-Rhys, R., & Jones, E. (2011). Social network sites and student–lecturer communication: An academic voice. *Journal of Further and Higher Education, 35*(2), 201–219. https://doi.org/10.1080/0309877X.2010.548596

Jones, N., & Corrigan, P. W. (2014). Understanding stigma. In P. W. Corrigan (ed.) *The stigma of disease and disability: Understanding causes and overcoming injustices* (pp. 9–34). Baltimore, MD: American Psychological Association.

Kamenetsky, S. B., Dimakos, C., Aslemand, A., Saleh, A., & Ali-Mohammed, S. (2016). Eliciting help without pity: The effect of changing media images on perceptions of disability. *Journal of Social Work in Disability and Rehabilitation, 15*(1), 1–21. https://doi.org/10.1080/1536710X.2016.1124251

Kaye, H. S., Jans, L. H., & Jones, E. C. (2011). Why don't employers hire and retain workers with disabilities? *Journal of Occupational Rehabilitation, 21*(4), 526–536. https://doi.org/10.1007/s10926-011-9302-8

Kelly, Y., Zilanawala, A., Booker, C., & Sacker, A. (2018). Social media use and adolescent mental health: Findings from the UK Millennium Cohort Study. *EClinicalMedicine, 6*, 59–68. https://doi.org/10.1016/j.eclinm.2018.12.005

Khan, R. (2021). *Domestic abuse policy guidance for UK universities.* Honour Abuse Research Matrix (HARM), University of Central Lancashire, UK. http://clok.uclan.ac.uk/37526/1/Domestic%20Abuse%20Policy%20Guidance%20for%20UK%20Universities%202021.pdf (accessed 11 January 2021).

Kinikoglu, C. N., & Can, A. (2021). Negotiating the different degrees of precarity in the UK academia during the COVID-19 pandemic. *European Societies, 23*(1), S817–S830. https://doi.org/10.1080/14616696.2020.1839670

Knight, M. T. D., Wykes, T., & Hayward, P. (2003). 'People don't understand': An investigation of stigma in schizophrenia using Interpretative Phenomenological Analysis (IPA). *Journal of Mental Health, 12*(3), 209–222. https://doi.org/10.1080/0963823031000118203

Korkmaz, N. C., Caviak, U., & Telci, E. A. (2011). Musculoskeletal pain, associated risk factors and coping strategies in school teachers. *Scientific Research and Essays, 6*(3), 649–657. https://doi.org/10.5897/SRE10.1064

Kowai-Bell, N., Guadagno, R. E., Little, T. E., & Ballew, J. L. (2012). Professors are people too: The impact of informal evaluations of professors on students and professors. *Social Psychology of Education, 15*, 337–351. https://doi.org/10.1007/s11218-012-9181-7

Krawczyk, M., & Smyk, M. (2016). Author's gender affects rating of academic articles: Evidence from an incentivized, deception-free laboratory experiment. *European Economic Review, 90*, 326–335. https://doi.org/10.1016/j.euroecorev.2016.02.017

Krukowski, R. A., Jagsi, R., & Cardel, M. I. (2020). Academic productivity differences by gender and child age in science, technology, engineering, and medicine faculty during the COVID-19 pandemic. *Journal of Women's Health, 30*(3), 341–347. https://doi.org/10.1089/jwh.2020.8710

Kuper, H., Banks, L. M., Bright, T., Davey, C., & Shakespeare, T. (2020). Disability-inclusive COVID-19 response: What it is, why it is important and what we can learn from the United Kingdom's response. *Wellcome Open Research, 5*(79), 1–5. https://doi.org/10.12688/wellcomeopenres.15833.1

La Monica, N. (2013). *Negotiating accommodations in academia: A matter of 'extra work'*. Paper presented at the International and Interdisciplinary Conference on Emotional Geographies at the University of Groningen, Netherlands, July.

Lampman, C., Phelps, A., Bancroft, S., & Beneke, M. (2009). Contrapower harassment in academia: A survey of faculty experience with student incivility, bullying and sexual attention. *Sex Roles, 60*(5/6), 331–346. https://doi.org/10.1007/s11199-008-9560-x

Landes, S. D., Turk, M. A., Formica, M. K., McDonald, K. E., & Stevens, J. D. (2020). COVID-19 outcomes among people with intellectual and developmental disability living in residential group homes in New York State. *Disability and Health Journal, 13*(4), 100969. https://doi.org/10.1016/j.dhjo.2020.100969

LaRocco, D. J., & Wilken, D. S. (2013). Universal Design for Learning: University faculty stages of concerns and levels of use. *Current Issues in Education, 16*(1). https://cie.asu.edu/ojs/index.php/cieatasu/article/view/1132 (accessed 11 January 2021).

Lathrop, D. (1995). Challenging perceptions, *Quill*, July/August, 37.

Law, C. L., Martinez, L. R., Ruggs, E. N., Hebl, M. R., & Akers, E. (2011). Transparency in the workplace: How the experiences of transsexual employees can be improved. *Journal of Vocational Behavior, 79*, 710–723. https://doi.org/10.1016/j.jvb.2011.03.018

Lawson, A., & Fouts, G. (2004). Mental illness in Disney animated films. *Canadian Journal of Psychiatry, 49*(5), 310–314. https://doi.org/10.1177/070674370404900506

Lazzerini, M., Barbi, E., Apicella, A., Marchetti, F., Cardinale, F., & Trobia, G. (2020). Delayed access of provision of care in Italy resulting from fear of COVID-19. *Lancet Child and Adolescent Health, 4*(5), e10–e11. https://doi.org/10.1016/S2352-4642(20)30108-5

Lea, J. (2010). *Political correctness and higher education: British and American perspectives*. New York: Routledge.

Leary, K. (1999). Passing, posing, and 'keeping it real'. *Constellations, 6*(1), 85–96. https://doi.org/10.1111/1467-8675.00122

Leckey, J., & Neill, N. (2001). Quantifying quality: The importance of student feedback. *Quality in Higher Education, 7*(1), 19–32. https://doi.org/10.1080/13538320120045058

Lee, S., Lee, M. T. Y., Chiu, M. Y. L., & Kleinman, A. (2005). Experience of social stigma by people with schizophrenia in Hong Kong. *British Journal of Psychiatry, 186*(2), 153–157. https://doi.org/10.1192/bjp.186.2.153

Lengnick-Hall, M. L., Gaunt, P. M., & Kulkani, M. (2008). Overlooked and underutilized: People with disabilities are an untapped human resource. *Human Resource Management, 47*(2), 255–273. https://doi.org/10.1002/hrm.20211

Leo, J., & Goodwin, D. (2016). Simulating others' realities: Insiders reflect on disability simulations. *Adapted Physical Activity Quarterly, 33*(2), 156–175. https://doi.org/10.1123/APAQ.2015-0031

Levinson, W., Kaufman, K., Clark, B., & Tolle, S. W. (1991). Mentors and role models for women in academic medicine. *Western Journal of Medicine, 154*(4), 423–426.

Libin, A., Schladen, M., Ljungberg, I., Tsai, B., Jacobs, S., Reinauer, K., Minnick, S., Spungen, M., & Groah, S. (2011). YouTube as an online disability self-management tool in persons with spinal cord injury. *Topics in Spinal Cord Injury Rehabilitation, 16*(3), 84–92. https://doi.org/10.1310/sci1603-84

Lindfelt, T., Ip, E. J., Gomez, A., & Barnett, M. J. (2018). The impact of work–life balance on intention to stay in academia: Results from a national survey of pharmacy faculty. *Research in Social and Administrative Pharmacy, 14*(4), 387–390. https://doi.org/10.1016/j.sapharm.2017.04.008

Llerena, A., Caceres, M. C., & Penas-Lledo, E. M. (2002). Schizophrenia stigma among medical and nursing undergraduates. *European Psychiatry, 17*(5), 298–299. https://doi.org/10.1016/S0924-9338(02)00672-7

Llewellyn, A., & Hogan, K. (2000). The use and abuse of models of disability. *Disability and Society, 15*(1), 157–165. https://doi.org/10.1080/09687590025829

Lockwood, P., Jordan, C. H., & Kunda, Z. (2002). Motivation by positive or negative role models: Regulatory focus determines who will best inspire us. *Journal of Personality and Social Psychology, 83*(4), 854–864. https://doi.org/10.1037//0022-3514.83.4.854

Lockwood, P., & Kunda, Z. (1997). Superstars and me: Predicting the impact of role models on the self. *Journal of Personality and Social Psychology, 73*(1), 91–103. https://doi.org/10.1037/0022-3514.73.1.91

Lok, P., & Crawford, J. (2004). The effect of organisational culture and leadership style on job satisfaction and organisational commitment: A cross-national comparison. *Journal of Management Development, 23*(4), 321–338. https://doi.org/10.1108/02621710410529785

Lourens, H. (2020). Supercripping the academy: The difference narrative of a disabled academic. *Disability and Society, 36*(8), 1205–1220. https://doi.org/10.1080/09687599.2020.1794798

Loveday, V. (2018). The neurotic academic: Anxiety, casualisation, and governance in the neoliberalising university. *Journal of Cultural Economy, 11*(2), 154–166. https://doi.org/10.1080/17530350.2018.1426032

Lund, E. M., & Ayers, K. B. (2020). Raising awareness of disabled lives and health care rationing during the COVID-19 pandemic. *Psychological Trauma: Theory, Research, Practice, and Policy, 12*(S1), S210–S211. https://doi.org/10.1037/tra0000673

Lyman, M., Beecher, M. E., Griner, D., Brooks, M., Call, J., & Jackson, A. (2016). What keeps students with disabilities from using accommodations in postsecondary education? A qualitative review. *Journal of Postsecondary Education and Disability, 29*(2), 123–140. http://www.ahead-archive.org/uploads/publications/JPED/jped292/JPED%2029_2_FullDocument.pdf (accessed 11 January 2021).

MacNell, L., Driscoll, A., & Hunt, A. N. (2015). What's in a name: Exposing gender bias in student ratings of teaching. *Innovative Higher Education, 40*(4), 291–303. https://doi.org/10.1007/s10755-014-9313-4

Madriaga, M. (2007). Enduring disablism: Students with dyslexia and their pathways into UK higher education and beyond. *Disability and Society, 22*(4), 399–412. https://doi.org/10.1080/09687590701337942

Major, B., & O'Brien, L. T. (2005). The social psychology of stigma. *Annual Review of Psychology, 56*, 393–421. https://doi.org/10.1146/annurev.psych.56.091103.070137

Mantilla, S., & Goggin, G. (2020). Thirty years of (in)visible disability in Australian television: *Home and Away*'s experiments with representation and inclusion. *Media International Australia, 174*(1), 39–48. https://doi.org/10.1177/1329878X19883890

Marchut, A. E., Pudans-Smith, K. K., Gietz, M. R., Andrews, J. F., & Clark, M. D. (2021). A case study of mentoring Deaf academics: The PAH! (Success) Academic Writing Retreat. *Creative Education, 12*, 176–192. https://doi.org/10.4236/ce.2021.121013

Marshak, L., Van Wieren, T., Ferrell, D. R., Swiss, L., & Dugan, C. (2009). Exploring barriers to college student use of disability services and accommodations. *Journal of Postsecondary Education and Disability, 22*(3), 151–165. https://www.ahead.org/professional-resources/publications/jped/archived-jped/jped-volume-22

Martin, J. M. (2010). Stigma and student mental health in higher education. *Higher Education Research and Development, 29*(3), 259–274. https://doi.org/10.1080/072943 60903470969

Martin, N. (2017). *Encouraging disabled leaders in higher education: Recognising hidden talents.* London: Leadership Foundation for Higher Education. https://openresearch.lsbu.ac.uk/item/8703y (accessed 11 January 2021).

Matcham, F., Rayner, L., Steer, S., & Hotopf, M. (2013). The prevalence of depression in rheumatoid arthritis: A systematic review and meta-analysis. *Rheumatology, 52*(12), 2136–2148. https://doi.org/10.1093/rheumatology/ket169

McKeon, B., Alpern, C. S., & Zager, D. (2013). Promoting academic engagement for college students with autism spectrum disorder. *Journal of Postsecondary Education and Disability, 26*(4), 353–366. https://files.eric.ed.gov/fulltext/EJ1026894.pdf (accessed 11 January 2021).

McMahon, B. T., & Shaw, L. R. (2005). Workplace discrimination and disability. *Journal of Vocational Rehabilitation, 23*(3), 137–143.

McNaron, T. A. H. (1997). *Poisoned ivy: Lesbian and gay academics confronting homophobia.* Philadelphia, PA: Temple University Press.

Melin, M., Astvik, W., & Bernhard-Oettel, C. (2014). New work demands in higher education: A study of the relationship between excessive workload, coping strategies and subsequent health among academic staff. *Quality in Higher Education, 20*(3), 290–308. https://doi.org/10.1080/13538322.2014.979547

Mellifont, D., Smith-Merry, J., Dickinson, H., Clifton, G. L. S., Ragen, J., Raffaele, M., & Williamson, P. (2019). The ableism elephant in the academy: A study examining academia as informed by Australian scholars with lived experience. *Disability and Society, 34*(7/8), 1180–1199. https://doi.org/10.1080/09687599.2019.1602510

Mercer-Mapstone, L., Dvorakova, S. L., Matthews, K. E., Abbot, S., Cheng, B., Felten, P., … & Swaim, K. (2017). A systematic literature review of students as partners in higher education. *International Journal for Students as Partners, 1*, 1–23. https://doi.org/10.15173/ijsap.v1i1.3119

Merchant, W., Read, S., D'Evelyn, S., Miles, C., & Williams, V. (2020). The insider view: Tackling disabling practices in higher education institutions. *Higher Education, 80*, 273–287. https://doi.org/10.1007/s10734-019-00479-0

Messiah University Code of Conduct (2021) https://www.messiah.edu/info/20854/additional_resources/3310/code_of_conduct_at_messiah_university (accessed 4 May 2021).

Miller, D. (2011). The dyslexic researcher: A call to broaden our portals. *Academy of Management Learning and Education, 10*(2), 340–350. https://doi.org/10.5465/amle.10.2.zqr340

Miller, J. (2019). Where does the time go? An academic workload case study at an Australian university. *Journal of Higher Education Policy and Management, 41*(6), 633–645. https://doi.org/10.1080/1360080X.2019.1635328

Mills, M. L. (2017). Invisible disabilities, visible service dogs: The discrimination of service dog handlers. *Disability and Society, 32*(5), 635–656. https://doi.org/10.1080/096 87599.2017.1307718

Mitra, S. (2006). The capability approach and disability. *Journal of Disability Policy Studies, 16*(4), 236–247. https://doi.org/10.1177/10442073060160040501

Mitra, S., Palmer, M., Kim, H., Mont, D., & Groce, N. (2017). Extra costs of living with a disability: A review and agenda for research. *Disability and Health Journal, 10*(4), 475–484. https://doi.org/10.1016/j.dhjo.2017.04.007

Mkumbo, K. (2014). Prevalence of and factors associated with work stress in academia in Tanzania. *International Journal of Higher Education, 3*(1), 1–11. https://doi.org/10.5430/ijhe.v3n1p1

Moore, S., & Kuol, N. (2005). A punitive bureaucratic tool or a valuable resource? Using student evaluations to enhance your teaching. In G. O'Neill, S. Moore, & B. McMullin (eds.) *Emerging issues in the practice of university learning and teaching* (pp. 141–148). Dublin: AISHE. http://citeseerx.ist.psu.edu/viewdoc/download;jsessionid=5BB55E712A3F1FA281DBFD28B9657B53?doi=10.1.1.489.6508&rep=rep1&type=pdf

Morgan, A. J., & Jorm, A. F. (2009). Recall of news stories about mental illness by Australian youth: Associations with help-seeking attitudes and stigma. *Australian and New Zealand Journal of Psychiatry*, *43*(9), 866–872. https://doi.org/10.1080/00048670903107567

Morgan, R., Hawkins, K., & Lundine, J. (2018). The foundation and consequences of gender bias in grant peer review processes. *Canadian Medical Association Journal*, *190*(16), E487–E488. https://doi.org/10.1503/cmaj.180188

Morris, D., & Turnbull, P. (2006). Clinical experiences of students with dyslexia. *Journal of Advanced Nursing*, *54*(2), 238–247. https://doi.org/10.1111/j.1365-2648.2006.03806.x

Morris, D. K., & Turnbull, P. A. (2007). The disclosure of dyslexia in clinical practice: Experiences of student nurses in the United Kingdom. *Nurse Education Today*, *27*(1), 35–42. https://doi.org/10.1016/j.nedt.2006.01.017

Moya, S., Prior, D., & Rodriguez-Perez, G. (2015). Performance-based incentives and the behavior of accounting academics: Responding to changes. *Accounting Education*, *24*(3), 208–232. https://doi.org/10.1080/09639284.2014.947092

Munir, F., Jones, D., Leka, S., & Griffiths, A. (2005). Work limitations and employer adjustments for employees with chronic illness. *International Journal of Rehabilitation Research*, *28*(2), 111–117. https://doi.org/10.1097/00004356-200506000-00003

Nario-Redmond, M. R., Kemerling, A. A., & Silverman, A. (2019). Hostile, benevolent, and ambivalent ableism: Contemporary manifestations. *Journal of Social Issues*, *75*(3), 726–756. https://doi.org/10.1111.josi.12337

Naslund, J. A., Aschbrenner, K. A., Marsch, L. A., & Bartels, S. J. (2016). The future of mental health care: Peer-to-peer support and social media. *Epidemiology and Psychiatric Sciences*, *25*(2), 113–122. https://doi.org/10.1017/S2045796015001067

National Association of Disabled Staff Networks (NADSN) (2020). *COVID-19 post-lockdown: Perspectives, implications and strategies for disabled staff*. https://www.nadsn-uk.org/covid-post-lockdown-perspectives-implications-and-strategies-for-disabled-staff-nadsn-position-paper/ (accessed 11 January 2021).

National Center on Disability and Journalism (2018). *Disability language style guide*. https://ncdj.org/style-guide/ (accessed 10 June 2020).

Nauta, M. M., & Kokaly, M. L. (2001). Assessing role model influences on students' academic and vocational decisions. *Journal of Career Assessment*, *9*(1), 81–99. https://doi.org/10.1177/106907270100900106

Nelson, J. A. (2000). The media role in building the disability community. *Journal of Mass Media Ethics*, *15*(3), 180–193. https://doi.org/10.1207/S15327728JMME1503-4

Oliveira, S. E., Esteves, F., & Carvalho, H. (2015). Clinical profiles of stigma experiences, self-esteem and social relationships among people with schizophrenia, depressive, and bipolar disorders. *Psychiatry Research*, *229*(1/2), 167–173. https://doi.org/10.1016/j.psychres.2015.07.047

Oliver, M. (1996). *Understanding disability: From theory to practice*. Basingstoke: Macmillan.

Olkin, R., Hayward, H., Abbene, M. S., & vanHeel, G. (2019). The experiences of microaggressions against women with visible and invisible disabilities. *Journal of Social Issues*, *75*(3), 757–785. https://doi.org/10.1111/josi.12342

Olsen, J., Griffiths, M., Soorenian, A., & Porter, R. (2020). Reporting from the margins: Disabled academics reflections on higher education. *Scandinavian Journal of Disability Research, 22*(1), 265–274. https://doi.org/10.16993/sjdr.670

Opini, B. M. (2010). A review of the participation of disabled persons in the labour force: The Kenyan context. *Disability and Society, 25*(3), 271–287. https://doi.org/10.1080/09687591003701181

Osborne, T. (2019). Not lazy, not faking: Teaching and learning experiences of university students with disabilities. *Disability and Society, 34*(2), 228–252. https://doi.org/10.1080/09687599.2018.1515724

Owen, P. R. (2012). Portrayals of schizophrenia by entertainment media: A content analysis of contemporary movies. *Psychiatric Services, 63*(7), 655–659. https://doi.org/10.1176/appi.ps.201100371

Pace, F., D'Urso, G., Zappulla, C., & Pace, U. (2019). The relation between workload and personal well-being among university professors. *Current Psychology, 40*, 3417–3424. https://doi.org/10.1007/s12144-019-00294-x

Paetzold, R. L., Garcia, M. F., Colella, A., Ren, L. R., del Carmen Triana, M., & Ziebro, M. (2008). Perceptions of people with disabilities: When is accommodation fair? *Basic and Applied Social Psychology, 30*(1), 27–35. https://doi.org/10.1080/01973530701665280

Parizeau, L., Shillington, L., Hawkins, R., Sultana, F., Mountz, A., Mullings, B., & Peake, L. (2016). Breaking the silence: A feminist call to action. *Canadian Geographer, 60*(2), 192–204. https://doi.org/10.1111/cag.12265

Park, D. S. (2020). The invisible university is COVID-19 positive. *Trends in Genetics, 36*(8), 543–544. https://doi.org/10.1016/j.tig.2020.05.010

Pfeiffer, D. (2001). The conceptualization of disability. In S. N. Barnatt & B. M. Altman (eds.) *Exploring theories and expanding methodologies: Where we are and where we need to go*. Research in Social Science and Disability (vol. 2, pp. 29–52). Bingley: Emerald Group Publishing.

Pfeiffer, D., & Kassaye, W. W. (1991). Student evaluations and faculty members with a disability. *Disability, Handicap and Society, 6*(3), 247–251. https://doi.org/10.1080/02674649166780281

Pirkis, J., & Francis, C. (2012). *Mental illness in the news and the information media: A critical review*. https://www.bpdcommunity.com.au/static/uploads/files/2012-mental-illness-in-the-media-critical-review-2012-wfquycqzzsru.pdf (accessed 10 June 2020).

Popovich, P. M., Scherbaum, C. A., Scherbaum, K. L., & Polinko, N. (2003). The assessment of attitudes toward individuals with disabilities in the workplace. *Journal of Psychology, 137*(2), 163–177. https://doi.org/10.1080/00223980309600606

Pritchard, G. (2010). Disabled people as culturally relevant teachers. *Journal of Social Inclusion, 1*(1), 43–51. https://doi.org/10.36251/josi.4

Prowse, S. (2009). Institutional construction of disabled students. *Journal of Higher Education Policy and Management, 31*(1), 89–96. https://doi.org/10.1080/13600800802559302

Raghavendra, P., Newman, L., Grace, E., & Wood, D. (2015). Enhancing social participation in young people with communication disabilities living in rural Australia: Outcomes of a home-based intervention for using social media. *Disability and Rehabilitation, 37*(17), 1576–1590. https://doi.org/10.3109/09638288.2015.1052578

Ragins, B. R. (2008). Disclosure disconnects: Antecedents and consequences of disclosing invisible stigmas across life domains. *Academy of Management Review, 33*(1), 194–215. https://doi.org/10.5465/amr.2008.27752724

Raimo, A., Devlin-Scherer, R., & Zinicola, D. (2002). Learning about teachers through film. *Educational Forum, 66*(4), 314–323. https://doi.org/10.1080/00131720208984850

Ralph, S., Capewell, C., & Bonnett, E. (2016). Disability hate crime: Persecuted for difference. *British Journal of Special Education*, *43*(3), 215–232. https://doi.org/10.1111/1467-8578.12139

Rao, D., Angell, B., Lam, C., & Corrigan, P. (2008). Stigma in the workplace: Employer attitudes about people with HIV in Beijing, Hong Kong, and Chicago. *Social Science and Medicine*, *67*(10), 1541–1549. https://doi.org/10.1016/j.socscimed.2008.07.024

Raphael, R. (1985). *The teacher's voice: A sense of who we are*. Portsmouth, NH: Heinemann.

Rasinski, H. M., & Czopp, A. M. (2010). The effect of target status on witnesses' reactions to confrontations of bias. *Basic and Applied Social Psychology*, *32*, 8–16. https://doi.org/10.1080/01973530903539754

Rauscher, L., & McClintock, J. (1996). Ableism curriculum design. In M. Adams, L. A. Bell, & P. Griffen (eds.) *Teaching for diversity and social justice* (pp. 198–231). New York: Routledge.

Rawlins, C. M. (2019). The ivory tower of academia and how mental health is often neglected. *Future Science OA*, *5*(4), FSO392. https://doi.org/10.4155/fsoa-2019-0032

Reason, R. D., Millar, E. A. R., & Scales, T. C. (2005). Toward a model of racial justice ally development. *Journal of College Student Development*, *46*, 530–546. https://doi.org/10.1353/csd. 2005.0054

Reece, E. A., Nugent, O., Wheeler, R. P., Smith, C. W., Hough, A. J., & Winter, C. (2008). Adapting industry-style business model to academia in a system of performance-based incentive compensation. *Academic Medicine*, *83*(1), 76–84. https://doi.org/10.1097/ACM.0b013e31815c6508

Rees, L., Robinson, P., & Shields, N. (2018). A major sporting event or an entertainment show? A content analysis of Australian television coverage of the 2016 Olympic and Paralympic games. *Sport in Society*, *21*(12), 1974–1989. https://doi.org/10.1080/17430437.2018.1445996

Rees, L., Robinson, P., & Shields, N. (2019). Media portrayal of elite athletes with disability: A systematic review. *Disability and Rehabilitation*, *41*(4), 374–381. https://doi.org/10.1080/09638288.2017.1397775

Reevy, G. M., & Deason, G. (2014). Predictors of depression, stress and anxiety among non-tenure track faculty. *Frontiers in Psychology*, *5*, 701. https://doi.org/10.3389/fpsyg.2014.00701

Regent University Code of Conduct (2021) https://www.regent.edu/admin/stusrv/docs/StudentHandbook.pdf (accessed 4 May 2021).

Reid, L. D. (2010). The role of perceived race and gender in the evaluation of college teaching on RateMyProfessors.com. *Journal of Diversity in Higher Education*, *3*(3), 137–152. https://doi.org/10.1037/a0019854

Resnick, P. J. (1984). The detection of malingered mental illness. *Behavioral Sciences and the Law*, *2*(1), 21–38. https://doi.org/10.1002/bsl.2370020104

Rich, S., Diaconescu, A. O., Griffiths, J. D., & Lankarany, M. (2020). Ten simple rules for creating a brand-new virtual academic meeting (even amid a pandemic). *PLoS Computational Biology*, *16*(12), e1008485. https://doi.org/10.1037/journal.pcbi.1008485

Richardson, J. T., & Wydell, T. N. (2003). The representation and attainment of students with dyslexia in UK higher education. *Reading and Writing*, *16*(5), 475–503. https://doi.org/10.1023/A:1024261927214

Riddell, S., & Weedon, E. (2014). Disabled students in higher education: Discourses of disability and the negotiation of identity. *International Journal of Educational Research*, *63*, 38–46. https://doi.org/10.1016/j.ijer.2013.02.008

Riddick, B. (2003). Experiences of teachers and trainee teachers who are dyslexic. *International Journal of Inclusive Education, 7*(4), 389–402. https://doi.org/10.1080/1360311032000110945

Rintamaki, L. S., Davis, T. C., Skripkauskas, S., Bennett, C. L., & Wolf, M. S. (2006). Social stigma concerns and HIV medication adherence. *AIDS Patient Care and STDs, 20*(5), 359–368. https://doi.org/10.1089/apc.2006.20.359

Roberts, P. (2007). Neoliberalism, performativity and research. *International Review of Education, 53*, 349–365. https://doi.org/10.1007/s11159-007-9049-9

Robertson, S. M., & Ne'eman, A. D. (2008). Autistic acceptance, the college campus, and technology: Growth of neurodiversity in society and academia. *Disability Studies Quarterly, 28*(4). https://doi.org/10.18061/dsq.v28i4.146

Robinson, S. A. (2015). Overcoming dyslexia with fortitude: One man's journey for an education. *Wisconsin English Journal, 57*(2), 36–48.

Roulestone, A., & Williams, J. (2014). Being disabled, being a manager: 'Glass partitions' and conditional identities in the contemporary workplace. *Disability and Society, 29*(1), 16–29. https://doi.org/10.1080/09687599.2013.764280

Roush, S. E., & Sharby, N. (2011). Disability reconsidered: The paradox of physical therapy. *Physical Therapy, 91*(12), 1715–1727. https://doi.org/10.2522/ptj.20100389

Russo, J., & Beresford, P. (2015). Between exclusion and colonisation: Seeking a place for mad people's knowledge in academia. *Disability and Society, 30*(1), 153–157. https://doi.org/10.1080/09687599.2014.957925

Ryder, D., & Norwich, B. (2019). UK higher education lecturers' perspectives of dyslexia, dyslexic students and related disability provision. *Journal of Research in Special Educational Needs, 19*(3), 161–172. https://doi.org/10.1111/1471-3802.12438

Sabagh, Z., Hall, N. C., & Saroyan, A. (2018). Antecedents, correlates and consequences of faculty burnout. *Educational Research, 60*(2), 131–156. https://doi.org/10.1080/00131881.2018.1461573

Safran, S. P. (2001). Movie images of disability and war: Framing history and political ideology. *Remedial and Special Education, 22*(4), 223–232. https://doi.org/10.1177/074193250102200406

Saks, E. R. (2008). *The center cannot hold: My journey through madness.* London: Hachette Books.

Saltes, N. (2020a). 'It's all about student accessibility. No one ever talks about teacher accessibility': Examining ableist expectations in academia. *International Journal of Inclusive Education.* https://doi.org/10.1080/13603116.2020.1712483

Saltes, N. (2020b). Disability barriers in academia: An analysis of disability accommodation policies for faculty at Canadian Universities. *Canadian Journal of Disability Studies, 9*(1), 53–90. https://doi.org/10.15353/cjds.v9i1.596

Sampson, F. (2003). Globalization and the inequality of women with disabilities. *Journal of Law and Equality, 2*(1) 16.

Sanchez, N. F., Rankin, S., Callahan, E., Ng, H., Holaday, L., McIntosh, K., Poll-Hunter, N., & Sanchez, J. P. (2015). LGBT trainee and health professional perspectives on academic careers: Facilitators and challenges. *LGBT Health, 2*(4), 346–356. https://doi.org/10.1089/lgbt.2015.0024

Sang, K., Powell, A., Finkel, R., & Richards, J. (2015). 'Being an academic is not a 9-5 job': Long working hours and the 'ideal worker' in UK academia. *Labour and Industry, 25*(3), 235–249. https://doi.org/10.1080/10301763.2015.1081723

Sapiro, V., & Campbell, D. (2018). Report on the 2017 APSA Survey on Sexual Harassment at Annual Meetings. *Political Science and Politics, 51*(1), 197–206. https://doi.org/10.1017/S1049096517002104

Sarju, J. P. (2021). Nothing about us without us – Towards a genuine inclusion of disabled scientists and science students post pandemic. *Chemistry: A European Journal, 27*(41), 10489–10494. https://doi.org/10.1002/chem.202100268

Sarrett, J. C. (2018). Autism and accommodations in higher education: Insights from the autism community. *Journal of Autism and Developmental Disorders, 48*(3), 679–693. https://doi.org/10.1007/s10803-017-3353-4

Sayles, J. N., Ryan, G. W., Silver, J. S., Sarkisian, C. A., & Cunningham, W. E. (2007). Experiences of social stigma and implications for healthcare among a diverse population of HIV positive adults. *Journal of Urban Health, 84*, 814. https://doi.org/10.1007/s11524-007-9220-4

Scarf, D., Zimmerman, H., Winter, T., Boden, H., Graham, S., Riordan, B. C., & Hunter, J. A. (2020). Association of viewing films *Joker* or *Terminator: Dark Fate* with prejudice toward individuals with mental illness. *JAMA Network Open, 3*(4), e203423. https://doi.org/10.1001/jamanetworkopen.2020.3423

Scheid, T. L. (2005). Stigma as a barrier to employment: Mental disability and the Americans with Disabilities Act. *International Journal of Law and Psychiatry, 28*(6), 670–690. https://doi.org/10.1016/j.ijlp.2005.04.003

Schell, L. A., & Duncan, M. (1999). A content analysis of CBS's coverage of the 1996 Paralympic Games. *Adapted Physical Activity Quarterly, 16*, 27–47. https://doi.org/10.1123/apaq.16.127

Schur, L. (2003). Barriers or opportunities? The causes of contingent and part-time work among people with disabilities. *Industrial Relations, 42*(4), 589–622. https://doi.org/10.1111/1468-232X.00308

Schur, L., Kruse, D., Blasi, J., & Blank, P. (2009). Is disability disabling in all workplaces? Workplace disparities and corporate culture. *Industrial Relations, 48*(3), 381–410. https://doi.org/10.1111/j.1468-232X.2009.00565.x

Schwartz, M. A., & Elder, B. C. (2018). Dialogue about disability praxis between a Deaf law professor and a hearing education. In M. S. Jeffress (ed.) *International perspectives on teaching with a disability*. New York: Routledge.

Scollay, P. A., Doucett, M., Perry, M., & Winterbottom, B. (1992). AIDS education of college students: The effect of an HIV-positive lecturer. *AIDS Education and Prevention, 4*(2), 160–171. https://doi.org/

Scully, J. L. (2020). Disability, disablism, and COVID-19 pandemic triage. *Journal of Bioethical Inquiry, 17*, 601–605. https://doi.org/10.1007/s11673-020-10005-y

Sen, A. K. (1985). *Commodities and capabilities* (vol. 7). Amsterdam: Elsevier.

Seropian, M. (2003). General concepts in full scale simulation: Getting started. *Anesthesia and Analgesia, 97*(6), 1695–1705. https://doi.org/10.1213/01.ANE.0000090152.91261.D9

Shah, M., & Nair, C. S. (2012). The changing nature of teaching and unit evaluations in Australian universities. *Quality Assurance in Education, 20*(3), 274–288. https://doi.org/10.1108/09684881211240321

Shah, S. (2005). *Career success of disabled high-flyers*. London: Jessica Kingsley.

Shakespeare, T., & Watson, N. (2001). The social model of disability: An outdated ideology? In S. N. Barnatt & B. M. Altman (eds.) *Exploring theories and expanding methodologies: Where we are and where we need to go*. Research in Social Science and Disability (vol. 2, pp. 9–28). Bingley: Emerald Group Publishing.

Shanks, L., Jason, L. A., Evans, M., & Brown, A. (2013). Cognitive impairments associated with CFS and POTS. *Frontiers in Physiology, 4*, 113. https://doi.org/10.3389/fphys.2013.00113

Shannon, C. D., Schoen, B., & Tansey, T. N. (2009). The effect of contact, context, and social power on undergraduate attitudes toward persons with disabilities. *Journal of Rehabilitation, 75*(4), 11–18.

Sharma, M., Yadav, K., Ydav, N., & Ferdinand, K. C. (2017). Zika virus pandemic: Analysis of Facebook as a social media health information platform. *American Journal of Infection Control*, *45*(3), 301–302. https://doi.org/10.1016/j.ajc.2016.08.022

Shaw, S. C. K., & Anderson, J. L. (2017). Doctors with dyslexia: A world of stigma, stonewalling and silence, still? *MedEdPublish*, *6*(1), 1–10. https://doi.org/10.15694/mep.2017.000029

Shelley-Egan, C. (2020). Testing the obligations of presence in academia in the COVID-19 era. *Sustainability*, *12*(16), 6350. https://doi.org/10.3390/su12166350

Sheridan, L., & Kotevski, S. (2014). University teaching with a disability: Student learnings beyond the curriculum. *International Journal of Inclusive Education*, *18*(11), 1162–1171. https://doi.org/10.1080/13603116.2014.881567

Shier, M., Graham, J. R., & Jones, M. E. (2009). Barriers to employment as experienced by disabled people: A qualitative analysis in Calgary and Regina, Canada. *Disability and Society*, *24*(1), 63–75. https://doi.org/10.1080/09687590802535485

Shore, C., & Wright, S. (1999). Audit culture and anthropology: Neo-liberalism in British higher education. *Journal of the Royal Anthropological Institute*, *5*(4), 557–575. https://doi.org/10.2307/2661148

Shpigelman, C. N., & Gill, C. J. (2014). Facebook use by persons with disabilities. *Journal of Computer-Mediated Communication*, *19*(3), 610–624. https://doi.org/10.1111/jcc4.12059

Sibitz, I., Unger, A., Woppmann, A., Zidek, T., & Amering, M. (2011). Stigma resistance in patients with schizophrenia. *Schizophrenia Bulletin*, *37*(2), 316–323. https://doi.org/10.1093/schbul/sbp048

Silva, C. F., & Howe, P. D. (2012). The (in)validity of supercrip representation of Paralympian athletes. *Journal of Sport and Social Issues*, *36*(2), 174–194. https://doi.org/10.1177/0193723511433865

Silverschanz, P., Cortina, L. M., Konik, J., & Magley, V. J. (2008). Slurs, snubs, and queer jokes: Incidence and impact of heterosexist harassment in academia. *Sex Roles*, *58*, 179–191. https://doi.org/10.1007/s11199-007-9329-7

Skinner, T. (2011). Dyslexia, mothering and work: Intersecting identities, reframing, 'drowning' and resistance. *Disability and Society*, *26*(2), 125–137. https://doi.org/10.1080/09687599.2011.543859

Smith, D. H., & Andrews, J. F. (2015). Deaf and hard of hearing faculty in higher education: Enhancing access, equity, policy, and practice. *Disability and Society*, *30*(10), 1521–1536. https://doi.org/10.1080/09687599.2015.1113160

Snyder, L. A., Carmichael, J. S., Blackwell, L. V., Cleveland, J. N., & Thornton, G. C. (2010). Perceptions of discrimination and justice among employees with disabilities. *Employee Responsibilities and Rights Journal*, *22*(1), 5–19. https://doi.org/10.1007/s10672-009-9107-5

Soliman, I., & Soliman, H. (1997). Academic workload and quality. *Assessment and Evaluation in Higher Education*, *22*(2), 135–157. https://doi.org/10.1080/0260293970220204

Solis, S. (2006). I'm 'coming out' as disabled, but I'm 'staying in' to rest: Reflecting on elected and imposed segregation. *Equity and Excellence in Education*, *39*(2), 146–153. https://doi.org/10.1080/10665680500534007

Solovieva, T. I., Dowler, D. L., & Walls, R. T. (2011). Employer benefits from making workplace accommodations. *Disability and Health Journal*, *4*(1), 39–45. https://doi.org/10.1016/j.dhjo.2010.03.001

Sousa, B. J., & Clark, A. M. (2017). Getting the most out of academic conference attendance: Five key strategies. *International Journal of Qualitative Methods*, *16*(1), 1–2. https://doi.org/10.1177/1609406917740441

Sprague, J., & Massoni, K. (2005). Student evaluations and gendered expectations: What we can't count can hurt us. *Sex Roles, 53*(11/12), 779–793. https://doi.org/10.1007/s11199-005-8292-4

Stanley, N., Ridley, J., Manthorpe, J., Harris, J., & Hurst, A. (2007). *Disclosing disability: Disabled students and practitioners in social work, nursing and teaching. A research study to inform the Disability Rights Commission's formal investigation into fitness standards*. http://clok.uclan.ac.uk/5099/1/disclosingdisabilityreport07.pdf (accessed 11 January 2021).

Steinberg, A. G., Iezzoni, L. I., Conill, A., & Stineman, M. (2002). Reasonable accommodations for medical faculty with disabilities. *Journal of the American Medical Association, 288*(24), 3147–3154. https://doi.org/10.1001/jama.288.24.3147

Stone, S. D., Crooks, V. A., & Owen, M. (2013). Going through the back door: Chronically ill academics' experiences as 'unexpected workers'. *Social Theory and Health, 11*(2), 151–174. https://doi.org/10.1057/sth.2013.1

Strindlund, L., Abrandt-Dahlgren, M., & Stahl, C. (2019). Employers' views on disability, employability, and labor market inclusion: A phenomenographic study. *Disability and Rehabilitation, 41*(24), 2910–2917. https://doi.org/10.1080/09638288.2018.1481150

Stuart, H. (2006). Media portrayal of mental illness and its treatments. *CNS Drugs, 20*(2), 99–106. https://doi.org/10.2165/00023210-200620020-00002

Swain, J., & French, S. (2000). Towards an affirmation model of disability. *Disability and Society, 15*(4), 569–582. https://doi.org/10.1080/09687590050058189

Swann, W. B. (1983). Self-verification: Bringing social reality into harmony with the self. In J. Suis & A. G. Greenwald (eds.) *Social psychological perspectives on the self* (vol. 2, pp. 33–56). Hillsdale, NJ: Lawrence Erlbaum.

Swann, W. B. (1987). Identity negotiation: Where two roads meet. *Journal of Personality and Social Psychology, 53*(6), 1038–1051. https://doi.org/10.1037/0022-3514.53.6.1038

Swetnam, L. A. (1992). Media distortion of the teacher image. *The Clearing House, 66*(1), 30–32. https://doi.org/10.1080/00098655.1992.9955921

Taylor, V., & Raeburn, N. C. (1995). Identity politics as high-risk activism: Career consequences for lesbian, gay, and bisexual sociologists. *Social Problems, 42*(2), 252–273. https://doi.org/10.2307/3096904

Thomas, A. (2000). Stability of Tringo's hierarchy of preference toward disability groups: 30 years later. *Psychological Reports, 86*(3), 1155–1156. https://doi.org/10.1177/003329410008600315.2

Time to Change (2014). *Making a drama out of a crisis*. London: Time to Change.

Timperley, C., Sutherland, K. A., Wilson, M., & Hall, M. (2020). He moana pukepuke: Navigating gender and ethnic inequality in early career academics' conference attendance. *Gender and Education, 32*(1), 11–26. https://doi.org/10.1080/09540253.2019.1633464

Tregaskis, C., & Goodley, D. (2005). Disability research by disabled and non-disabled people: Towards a relational methodology of research production. *International Journal of Social Research Methodology, 8*(5), 363–374. https://doi.org/10.1080/13645570500402439

Tucker, B. (2014). Student evaluation surveys: Anonymous comments that offend or are unprofessional. *Higher Education, 68*(3), 347–358. https://doi.org/10.1007/s10734-014-9716-2

Tucker, F., & Horton, J. (2019). 'The show must go on!' Fieldwork, mental health and wellbeing in Geography, Earth and Environmental Sciences. *Area, 51*, 84–93. https://doi.org/10.1111/area.12437

Tuinamuana, K. (2016). The work of the teacher-educator in Australia: Reconstructing the 'superhero' performer/academic in an audit culture. *Asia-Pacific Journal of Teacher Education, 44*(4), 333–347. https://doi.org/10.1080/1359866X.2016.1194369

van Hees, V., Moyson, T., & Roeyers, H. (2015). Higher education experiences of students with autism spectrum disorder: Challenges, benefits and support needs. *Journal of Autism and Developmental Disorders, 45*(6), 1673–1688. https://doi.org/10.1007/s10803-014-2324-2

Vaughan, C., Khaw, S., Katsikis, G., Wheeler, J., Ozge, J., Kasidis, V., & Moosad, L. (2019). 'It is like being put through a blender': Inclusive research in practice in an Australian university. *Disability and Society, 34*(7/8), 1224–1240. https://doi.org/10.1080/09687599.2019.1603103

Vickers, M. H. (1997). Life at work with 'invisible' chronic illness (ICI): The 'unseen', unspoken, unrecognized dilemma of disclosure. *Journal of Workplace Learning, 9*(7), 240–252. https://doi.org/10.1108/13665629710190040

Vincent, A., Whipple, M. O., & Rhudy, L. M. (2016). Fibromyalgia flares: A qualitative analysis. *Pain Medicine, 17*(3), 463–468. https://doi.org/10.1111/pme.12676

Waaijer, C. J. F., Belder, R., Sonneveld, H., van Bochove, C. A., & van der Weijden, I. C. (2017). Temporary contracts: Effect on job satisfaction and personal lives of recent PhD graduates. *Higher Education, 74*(2), 321–339. https://doi.org/10.1007/s10734-016-0050-8

Wahl, O. (2003). Depictions of mental illnesses in children's media. *Journal of Mental Health, 12*(3), 249–258. https://doi.org/10.1080/0963823031000118230

Walker, A. (1996). *The same river twice*. New York: Washington Square Press.

Waterfield, B., Beagan, B., & Weinberg, M. (2018). Disabled academics: A case study in Canadian universities. *Disability and Society, 33*(3), 327–348. https://doi.org/10.1080/09687599.2017.1411251

Watson, N. (2002). Well, I know this is going to sound very strange to you, but I don't see myself as a disabled person: Identity and disability. *Disability and Society, 17*(5), 509–527. https://doi.org/10.1080/09687590220148496

Wearden, A. J., & Appleby, L. (1996). Research on cognitive complaints and cognitive functioning in patients with chronic fatigue syndrome (CFS): What conclusions can we draw? *Journal of Psychosomatic Research, 41*(3), 197–211. https://doi.org/10.1016/0022-3999(96)00131-6

Westine, C. D., Oyarzun, B., Ahlgrim-Delzell, L., Casto, A., Okraski, C., Park, G., Person, J., & Steele, L. (2019). Familiarity, current use, and interest in Universal Design for Learning among online university instructors. *International Review of Research in Open and Distributed Learning, 20*(5), 20–41. https://doi.org/10.19173/irrodl.v20i5.4258

White, S. W., Ollendick, T. H., & Bray, B. C. (2011). College students on the autism spectrum: Prevalence and associated problems. *Autism, 15*(6), 683–701. https://doi.org/10.1177/1362361310393363

Williams, J. (2011). *What can disabled academics' career experiences offer to studies of organization?* Doctoral thesis. Northumbria University. https://nrl.northumbria.ac.uk/4450/

Williams, J., & Mavin, S. (2015). Impairment effects as a career boundary: A case study of disabled academics. *Studies in Higher Education, 40*(1), 123–142. https://doi.org/10.1080/03075079.2013.818637

Wilson-Kovacs, D., Ryan, M. K., Haslam, A., & Rabinovich, A. (2008). 'Just because you can get a wheelchair in the building doesn't necessarily mean that you can still participate': Barriers to the career advancement of disabled professionals. *Disability and Society, 23*(7), 705–717. https://doi.org/10.1080/09687590802469198

Woodburn, D., & Ruderman, J. (2016). Op-Ed: Why are we OK with disability drag in Hollywood? *Los Angeles Times*, 11 July. https://www.latimes.com/opinion/op-ed/la-oe-woodburn-ruderman-disability-stats-tv-20160711-snap-story.html (accessed 10 June 2020).

Woodcock, K., Rohan, M. J., & Campbell, L. (2007). Equitable representation of deaf people in mainstream academia: Why not? *Higher Education, 53*(3), 359–379. https://doi.org/10.1007/s10734-005-2428-x

Woods, J. D. (1994). *The corporate closet*. New York: Free Press.

Woolston, C. (2018). Feeling overwhelmed by academia? You are not alone. *Nature, 557*(7706), 129–131. https://doi.org/10.1038/d41586-018-04998-1

Zaussinger, S., & Terzieva, B. (2018). Fear of stigmatization among students with disabilities in Austria. *Social Inclusion, 6*(4), 182–193. https://doi.org/10.17645/si.v6i4.1667

Zhao, Y., & Zhang, J. (2017). Consumer health information seeking in social media: A literature review. *Health Information and Libraries Journal, 34*(4), 268–283. https://doi.org/10.1111/hir.12192

Index

Accessible Buildings 25, 37, 39, 56, 81, 84, 87, 89, 96–97, 99
Activism and Campaigns 1, 5, 6, 7, 9, 10, 11, 13, 17, 18, 19–20, 28–29, 73, 99, 101
Advertising 3–4
Aesthetics, *see* Appearance
Affirmation Model 10–11
Anxiety, 27, 28, 35, 40, 49, 50, 51, 56, 58, 61–63, 65, 67, 75, 94, 102 *see also* Mental Health
Appearance 3, 8, 18
Arthritis, *see* Musculoskeletal Disorders
Athlete, *see* Sport
Autism 56–58, 70
Autoethnography 41, 63, 68

Biological Model, *see* Medical Model
Blame 15, 19, 20, 66
Blind, *see* Sensory Impairment

Campaigns, *see* Activism and Campaigns
Capability Model 10–11
Cerebral Palsy 2, 4, 13, 74
Charity 1, 4
Children, *see* Parenting
Chronic Pain, *see* Pain
Competence 17, 21, 24, 26, 36, 47–48, 55, 63, 71, 74, 78, 81, 82
Conferences 11–12, 26, 31, 34, 37–38, 56, 57, 60, 64, 66, 72, 84, 87, 88, 93, 95–98, 101, 102, 103
Contested Conditions 66–67, 80, 91
Coping 37, 38, 59, 60, 62, 63, 67, 81
Covering, *see* Passing
COVID-19 6, 40–42, 44, 57, 62, 64, 67–68, 98, 101–103
Creativity 32, 45, 60, 86, 90

Deaf, *see* Sensory Impairment
Deficit 11, 19, 47, 99, 100
Depression, 20, 22, 27, 43, 51, 56, 61–63, 65, 74, 75 *see also* Mental Health

Diagnosis 2, 4, 6, 8, 11, 39, 44, 48, 49, 56, 79, 80, 91–92, 94, 96, 99
Disability Drag 2–3
Disability Pride 73
Disabled Staff Networks 45, 92, 98–99, 103, 104
Disabled Students 15, 21, 24, 25, 36, 38, 42, 46, 51, 56–61, 70, 71–73, 75–76, 77, 78, 80, 84, 86, 87–88, 89–90, 94, 95, 99, 100
Dyslexia 21, 52, 58–61, 71, 76, 84, 87, 90

Energy Limiting Conditions, *see* Fatigue
Euthanasia 2, 9

Facebook, *see* Social Media
Faking Disability 3, 23, 76–80
Fatigue, 10, 16–17, 18, 23, 27, 34, 43–44, 48, 51, 61, 63, 64, 65–67, 74, 80, 84, 85, 89, 91, 94, 97, 98, 102
Fieldwork 38, 67, 94
Fluctuating Conditions 23, 77–78, 79–80, 81, 90, 100

Gender, 10, 12, 15, 18–19, 24, 28, 40, 52, 62, 64, 69–70, 72, 78, 95, 98, 104
Giroux 32–33
Goffman 16–17, 51

Harassment, *see* Violence
Hearing loss, *see* Sensory Impairment
Hero, 1, 6, 13 *see also* Supercrip Narrative
Hierarchy of Disability 13, 65, 73, 91, 100
HIV/AIDS 20–21
Home Working, *see* Remote Working
Honour Codes 29

Identity, disabled 1, 6, 7, 11, 12, 16–18, 34, 43–46, 48–50, 54, 63, 73–74, 92
Inspiration porn, *see* Supercrip narrative
Interview, *see* Recruitment
Isolation 4, 6, 10, 17, 21, 26, 28, 38, 50, 52, 62, 102

Job Satisfaction 30, 32, 35, 72
Job Security 20, 22, 25, 31, 33, 35, 36, 37, 40, 42, 47, 53, 61, 85–86

Language 4, 7–8, 26, 54, 86, 92
Leadership, *see* Management
Legislation 3, 9, 16, 103
Legitimacy, *see* Contested Conditions, Hierarchy of Disability, Malingering

Magazines 5
Malingering, *see* Faking Disability
Management 21, 25, 27, 38–39, 43, 47, 48, 49, 50, 55, 71, 83, 84–85, 86, 89, 90–91, 93, 96, 99, 100, 103
Media Representation of Disability 1–7, 13–14, 15, 20, 48, 66, 78, 101
Media Representation of Teachers and Academics 14–15, 53, 101
Medical Model 8–9, 10, 11, 39, 100
Medical Practitioners and Professionals 5, 7, 8–9, 11, 14, 20, 22, 43, 44, 58–59, 66, 75, 79–80, 91–92, 94
Mental Health *see* Anxiety, Autism, Depression, Schizophrenia
Mentoring 12, 21, 57, 71–73, 86–87, 98
Metrics, *see* Performance Metrics
Models of Disability 1, 8–11, 12, 39, 77, 100
Musculoskeletal disorders 43, 45, 63–65, 102

Neurodiversity, 2, 60, 84 *see also* Autism, Dyslexia

Occupational Health 28–39, 41, 50, 63, 91
Othering 13, 47
Overcoming Disability 2, 9, 13–14, 15, 59, 73

Pain 10, 47, 53, 74, 91,
Pandemic, *see* COVID-19
Paralympic and Olympic Games 2, 13–14
Parenting 11, 14, 15, 34, 40, 60, 62, 71
Part-Time Employment or Study 22, 66, 78, 85–86, 87–88
Passing 16, 23, 43, 49–50, 62, 63
Patient and Service User Involvement
Performance Metrics 30, 31, 32, 33, 88–89
Precarious Working, *see* Job Security

Productivity, 22, 23, 31, 32, 35–36, 40, 42, 46, 47, 61, 62, 83–84, 85–86, 91, 100 *see also* Performance Metrics, Publication, Workload
Promotion 25, 26, 27, 29, 33, 37, 39, 40, 69, 72, 84–85, 86, 87, 98
Publication, Research 31, 40, 42, 60, 63, 72, 84, 86–87, 96

Recruitment 16, 26, 29, 40, 45–46, 71, 82, 84, 86, 91
Rehabilitation and Treatment 2, 5, 8–9, 11, 17, 20–21, 35, 38, 41, 67, 91, 93, 94, 100, 102, 103
Remote Working, 34, 41–42, 44–45, 48, 57, 65, 66, 67–68, 101–103 *see also* COVID-19
Research Funding 19, 31, 37, 67, 87–88
Research Outputs, *see* Conferences, Research Funding, Publication
Retention 22, 23, 40, 69, 83, 91, 100
Role Models 71–73, 75–76

Self-Esteem 20, 46, 60, 73
Self-Stigma 17–18, 20 *see also* Disability Pride
Sensory Impairment 8, 22, 27, 38, 70, 80, 86–87, 90, 97
Schizophrenia 4, 19–20, 27
Sexual Orientation 12, 28–29, 46, 69
Sickness Absence 17, 34, 38, 55, 63, 77, 100
Social Media 5–7, 26, 37, 53, 101
Social Model 8, 9–10, 100
Sport 2, 13–14, 52
Stereotypes, 1–2, 4–5, 6, 7–8, 13–15, 17–21, 24, 26, 28, 36, 58, 62, 69–70, 71, 74, 81, 94, 99, 102
Stress 26–27, 28, 33, 35, 40, 46, 49, 50, 56, 61, 62, 65, 67
Student Evaluations 35, 69–71, 103
Supercrip Narrative 1–2, 13–14, 15

Tenure, *see* Job Security
Threat, *see* Violence
Training 22, 23, 39, 59, 60–61, 80–82, 93, 99–101, 103
Travel 6, 12, 34, 37, 38, 64, 79, 81, 87, 93, 96, 101–102
Twitter, *see* Social Media

Union 17
Universal Design 89, 96, 98

Violence and Aggression 1–2, 5, 18, 20, 21, 26, 28–29, 36, 46, 51, 62, 57, 78, 95–96

Wheelchair Use, 3, 7, 9, 13, 16, 18–19, 23, 28, 70, 75, 76, 78, 80–82, 90, 97, 98
Workload 14, 15, 24, 27, 28, 33–35, 38–39, 47, 55, 64, 83–85, 101
Workload Allocation Models 35, 84